MIGRANTS WHO CARE

CAREWORK IN A CHANGING WORLD

Amy Armenia, Mignon Duffy, and Kim Price-Glynn, Series Editors

The rise of scholarly attention to care has accompanied greater public concern about aging, health care, child care, and labor in a global world. Research on care is happening across disciplines—in sociology, economics, political science, philosophy, public health, social work, and others—with numerous research networks and conferences developing to showcase this work. Care scholarship brings into focus some of the most pressing social problems facing families today. To study care is to also study the future of work, as issues of carework are intertwined with the forces of globalization, technological development, and the changing dynamics of the labor force. Care scholarship also is at the cutting edge of intersectional analyses of inequality, as carework often is at the very core of understanding gender, race, migration, age, disability, class, and international inequalities.

Mignon Duffy, Amy Armenia, and Kim Price-Glynn, eds., *From Crisis to Catastrophe: Care, COVID, and Pathways to Change*

Fumilayo Showers, *Migrants Who Care: West Africans Working and Building Lives in U.S. Health Care*

MIGRANTS WHO CARE

West Africans Working and Building Lives in U.S. Health Care

FUMILAYO SHOWERS

R

RUTGERS UNIVERSITY PRESS

New Brunswick, Camden, and Newark, New Jersey
London and Oxford

Rutgers University Press is a department of Rutgers, The State University of New Jersey, one of the leading public research universities in the nation. By publishing world-wide, it furthers the University's mission of dedication to excellence in teaching, scholarship, research, and clinical care.

Library of Congress Cataloging-in-Publication Data
Names: Showers, Fumilayo, author.
Title: Migrants who care : West Africans working and building lives in U.S. health care / Fumilayo Showers.
Description: New Brunswick : Rutgers University Press, [2023] | Series: Carework in a changing world | Includes bibliographical references and index.
Identifiers: LCCN 2022057007 | ISBN 9781978828988 (paperback) | ISBN 9781978828995 (cloth) | ISBN 9781978829008 (epub) | ISBN 9781978829015 (pdf)
Subjects: LCSH: Medical personnel, Foreign—United States. | West Africans—Migrations—United States.
Classification: LCC R697.F6 S53 2023 | DDC 610.69089/966073—dc23/eng/20230505
LC record available at https://lccn.loc.gov/2022057007

A British Cataloging-in-Publication record for this book is available from the British Library.

♾ The paper used in this publication meets the requirements of the American National Standard for Information Sciences—Permanence of Paper for Printed Library Materials, ANSI Z39.48-1992.

rutgersuniversitypress.org

To my parents, Moses and Adeliza, for imparting a love of learning; and to my aunt, Violet, whose journey to America and career successes made my own possible

CONTENTS

CONTENTS

ABBREVIATIONS

ACA	Affordable Care Act
BSN	bachelor of science in nursing
CGFNS	Commission on Graduates of Foreign Nursing Schools
CNA	certified nursing assistant
DDS	Department of Disability Services
DNP	doctor of nursing practice
DOH	Department of Health
DON	director of nursing
DSP	direct support professional
FNP-C	family nurse practitioner-clinical care
HHA	home health aide
ISP	Individual Support Plan
LPN	licensed practical nurse
MSN	master of science in nursing
NCLEX	National Council Licensure Examination
NCLEX-PN	National Council Licensure Examination for Practical or Vocational Nurses
NCLEX-RN	National Council Licensure Examination for Registered Nurses
NP	nurse practitioner
PPE	personal protective equipment
PPP	Payment Protection Program
QIDP	qualified intellectual disability support professional
RN	registered nurse

MIGRANTS WHO CARE

INTRODUCTION

Arthurlina Stevens is a fifty-year-old nurse from Sierra Leone, West Africa, who has lived and worked in the suburbs of Washington, DC, for twenty years. Arthurlina is a tall, imposing woman with a broad and welcoming smile. Her career in health care began when she trained as a nurse in her homeland after completing her high school education. Her professional trajectory was, however, halted when a civil war in Sierra Leone drove her to the United States. Her Sierra Leonean friends in the United States helped her with information about the job market, and her extended family provided a place for her to stay when she first arrived. She re-trained as a nurse while working as a certified nursing assistant (CNA[1]) because U.S. employers would not accept the nursing credentials she had earned from home. While proud of her accomplishments in the U.S. labor market, she also remembered the difficulties she faced when she first arrived. Working as a CNA meant low pay and back-breaking duties as she cared for vulnerable older adults in nursing homes. Despite these difficulties, Arthurlina persevered, attending night classes after working excruciatingly long daytime hours. She earned both bachelor's and master's degrees in nursing, and at the time of our meeting, she was working as a nursing director in a nursing home.

Albert Kamara, also a middle-aged Sierra Leonean immigrant, has, similarly, achieved a supervisory role in health care. His job involves supervising a team of residential care staff and coordinating medical, legal, and other services for his care recipients who suffer from physical and intellectual disabilities. Albert is a popular member of staff in a health care provision company owned and managed by Sierra Leonean immigrants. He has a very professional demeanor, and is always impeccably dressed in a blazer, crisp work shirt, and nicely pressed trousers. He exudes a quiet dignity, and it is obvious that the junior staff look up to him and that his employers value him. Albert was a university lecturer in his native Sierra Leone prior to migration and held a master's degree. After migrating to the United States as a working-age adult, he first sought employment as an economist but was unsuccessful. Albert explained that fellow Sierra Leonean immigrants encouraged him to join the care workforce and made the connections that landed him the job he now holds. He had worked with his present company for fifteen years when we spoke and had risen through the ranks, starting as a direct support professional[2] then becoming a qualified intellectual disability professional[3] responsible for supervising the paraprofessional staff in the residential homes operated by the company.

Rose Asamoah, by contrast, came to the United States before starting her career. Now in her thirties, she migrated to the United States from Ghana, West Africa, in her late teens to pursue undergraduate education at a small, private liberal arts college. After graduating from college in the United States with a major in psychology, she abandoned a plan to attend medical school because she recognized her grades would make it difficult for her to gain admission. She researched dentistry school and pharmacy school before deciding on nursing school, against the wishes of her family in Ghana, who perceived nursing as a career track not befitting her privileged background. She graduated from a top nursing program and was working as a registered nurse in a hospital when I interviewed her.

This book is about immigrants like Arthurlina, Albert, and Rose, who leave their homes in West Africa for varied reasons, migrate through various channels and provisions in immigration law, and become absorbed into the U.S. health care labor market. Their stories provide a glimpse into a labor phenomenon that, while still largely unnoticed in the scholarly and popular discourses on immigration in the United States, has become more visible in nursing homes, hospitals, and private homes in major cities. This is the reality of immigrants, from diverse racial, ethnic, and national backgrounds, who become produced, repackaged, and deployed as health care workers after migration. In the United States, they care for the sick, frail older adults, and physically or intellectually disabled care recipients, and they work in hospitals, institutional care settings such as nursing homes, and private homes. This book unearths this immigrant story, focusing on a sample of African immigrant women and men from five nations (Ghana, Nigeria, Liberia, Sierra Leone, and Cameroon) who live and work in the Washington, DC, metropolitan area. Research subjects worked as home health aides, certified nursing assistants, qualified disability support professionals, licensed practical and registered nurses, and as formal and informal labor recruiters and brokers for jobs in the health industry.

I argue that the experiences of African immigrants reveal a case of immigrant labor incorporation, where individuals become health care workers due to discrimination in other sectors of the primary labor market, structural gendered demands in the care industry, and racialization[4] that constructs immigrants of color as ideal for low-wage direct care work[5] and unattractive specializations within professional health care occupations. They are aided in their migratory journeys by coethnics already settled in the United States, many of whom also work in nursing, home/elder care, and disability support. This concentration in various sectors in health care exemplifies what immigration scholars call an immigrant niche of employment; that is, when an immigrant group is overrepresented in an industry or line of work relative to the group's proportion in the host country or their share of a total labor force (Eckstein and Peri 2018; Hamilton et al. 2018; Light and Gold 2000; Waldinger 1994, 1996; Waldinger and Lichter 2003) or when an immigrant group's social networks extend to multiple parts of an industry rather than a single one (Poros 2011).

While often starting out at the base of labor hierarchies in health care as paraprofessional workers such as nursing aides, home health aides, and direct support professionals and encountering racialized hierarchies and workplace racism in various occupational segments, many Black African immigrant professionals have been upwardly mobile, moving on to professional careers in nursing or positions of increased authority in disability support and elder care. Some have opened businesses in health and long-term care, hiring mostly other West Africans. Their ability to adjust, cope, and attain upward social and economic mobility is shaped by gender, social class, immigration status, access to social capital deployed within immigrant social networks and businesses, and occupational context, so that African immigrants working in varying contexts have different experiences.

Ultimately, this book tells the very real human story of an immigrant group who have surmounted tremendous obstacles to carve out a labor market niche in health care, providing some of the most essential and intimate aspects of care labor to the most vulnerable members of society.

To set the context for the discussion of their roles in care occupations, it is important to understand who these immigrants to the United States are and how their increasing presence is changing the racial and social contours of American life. In the next section, I provide a demographic portrait of recent African immigrants.

AFRICAN IMMIGRATION TO THE UNITED STATES SINCE 1980

The migration of Sub-Saharan Africans to the United States has increased since 1980, when the entire African-born population in the United States was less than 200,000 people (Echevarria-Estrada and Batalova 2019; McCabe 2012). By 2018, there were slightly over 2 million people born in Sub-Saharan Africa living in the country. (Echevarria-Estrada and Batalova 2019). Between 2010 and 2018, the Sub-Saharan African immigrant population increased by 52 percent, significantly surpassing the 12 percent growth rate of the overall immigrant population over that same time (Echevarria-Estrada and Batalova 2019). As the data suggests, Sub-Saharan Africans are one of the fastest growing immigrant groups in the United States (Anderson 2015; Halter and Showers Johnson 2014; Hamilton 2019; Imoagene 2017).

The increasing numbers of voluntary immigrants from Africa has given rise to a burgeoning literature on what has been termed the "new African Diaspora" (Gordon 1998; Konadu-Agyemang and Takyi 2006). In 2015, West Africa was the leading region of birth of African immigrants, comprising about 45 percent of the total African immigrant population in the United States (Zong and Batalova 2017). The top sending countries from West Africa are Nigeria, Ghana, Liberia, Cape Verde, and Sierra Leone (Zong and Batalova 2017). Sub-Saharan Africans are concentrated in large metropolitan areas, with large populations in Texas (Harris county), New York (Bronx county), Maryland (Prince George's and Montgomery counties), and Minnesota (Hennepein county) (Lorenzi and Batalova 2022).

A few studies have explored the labor market experiences of recent African immigrants to North America within specific occupational niches. Sociologist John Arthur (2009) reported the presence of African immigrant women in agriculture, meatpacking, construction, and elder care. Historians Marilyn Halter and Violet Showers Johnson found that West African immigrants are prevalent in the service economy—"in hospitality services, in the health care industry, where they work as nurses, nursing assistants, orderlies, or respiratory and lab assistants, or in transportation related jobs such as taxi drivers and airport porters—with the men also working in construction and extraction" (Halter and Showers Johnson 2014, 25). Regarding health care professions, they noted that a third of African women living in the United States were working in health care jobs in 2009, and that African men and women were more likely than other U.S. immigrants to work in health care (Halter and Showers Johnson 2014, 25–26). A 2012 study noted that African men and women workers were more likely to report holding jobs as health care practitioners and in other health care support occupations. Indeed, "compared to male immigrants overall, African-born male workers were more likely to report working as health care practitioners and in other health care support occupations" (McCabe 2012). More recent accounts show that though a small share of the total immigrant population (4.5 percent), Africans make up 12 percent of the immigrant share of the health care labor force (Batalova 2020; Echevarria-Estrada and Batalova 2019). Within health care occupations, African immigrants are more likely to work as registered nurses and in health care support occupations such as home health aides, certified nursing assistants, and disability support professionals (Batalova 2020).

This growing presence of Africans in the United States and their concentrations in health care, in both professional (nursing) and paraprofessional sectors of the industry (disability support, nursing, and home care support) motivated the writing of this book. I build on the work of historian Martha Donkor (2017) and anthropologist Cati Coe (2019), who have documented the lived experiences of African immigrant elder care workers caring for a mostly white and affluent population. Their accounts have been replete with themes of exploitation, victimhood, and servitude within a particular segment of the long-term care industry: elder care in home settings. These accounts have also portrayed these care jobs as "dead-end" jobs with very little room for upward mobility and financial security. Casting a wider lens and focusing on West Africans across the continuum of professional levels in institutional and home care, I argue that low-level health care positions can and do lead to some opportunities for upward mobility. Many of the individuals in this book started out at the bottom of the labor market in the care industry but were able to achieve some mobility within the field and across occupational segments. A few were even able to open businesses that tapped into a racialized market for care and capitalized on the labor of their coethnics.

This book charts the macro-level processes through which these immigrants have become concentrated in various roles across the spectrum of professional levels in the health industry, caring not only for white patients but also for a significant number of African American care recipients. I extend my analysis beyond care in home settings to explore workers' experiences in institutional care settings such as hospitals, nursing homes, and residential and day care settings for adult care recipients. While acknowledging the challenges of the field, I also show how research subjects enact individual strategies at the micro-level and create and deploy social capital within their transnational social networks to find economic mobility, success, and meaning in care jobs. I present these immigrants as agents rather than victims and demonstrate their "agentic maneuvers" (Banerjee 2022) in carving paths of mobility within health care occupations. In telling this story, I highlight African immigrants' contributions to the care industry specifically and U.S. society more broadly.

THE CRISIS OF CARE IN THE UNITED STATES AND IN THE GLOBAL ECONOMY

The focus on care occupations in this book is important, because worker shortages and rising demands have raised the question as to who will provide care for the increasing numbers of older adult as well as disabled populations in need of long-term care in the United States and other advanced economies (Boris and Klein 2012; Ehrenreich and Hochschild 2004; Glenn 2010; Gottfried and Chun 2018; Stacey 2011). As members of the baby boom generation age and require care and current health care workers in that generation are increasingly likely to retire, U.S. health care institutions are projected to face future staffing challenges (Kingma 2005; Squires and Beltran-Sanchez 2013). Further, geographic distances between adult children and their parents have increased, while women have entered the formal workforce in greater numbers (Buch 2018; Duffy 2005; Harrington-Meyer 2000; Stacey 2011). Neoliberal ideology drives U.S. federal and state governments' moves to deinstitutionalize and privatize care for vulnerable older adults and adults with intellectual and physical disabilities, resulting in the increasing need for both paid health care and reproductive care in the home (Batalova 2020; Buch 2018; Coe 2019; Kingma 2005; Wingfield 2019). These demographic, economic, and social changes have translated into a growth in the personal home care industry (Batalova 2020; Boris and Klein 2012; Duffy et al. 2015; Glenn 2010; Stacey 2011).[6] Medical advancement and innovations, which allow for more individuals to live longer with chronic health problems, increase demand for professional and paraprofessional health care workers in institutional and long-term care settings such as hospitals and nursing homes (Batalova 2020; Buerhaus et al. 2003; Duffy et al. 2015; Ong and Azores 1994).[7]

The growth in health care occupations, including home health care and institutional care, has led to an overall increase in the number of foreign-born[8] health care workers, since the supply of native-born health care workers has failed to meet the growing demand (Batalova 2020; Altorjai and Batalova 2017).[9] The literature attuned to matters of gender and global migration has, consequently, paid increasing attention to the migration of professional health care workers from the global south to fill these shortages in health care institutions in the United States and other nations of the global north (Choy 2003; Dovlo 2006; George 2005; Guevarra 2010; Kingma 2005; Ong and Azores 1994; Ortiga 2017, 2018; Rodriguez 2010). The literature on the migration of professional health care workers exists alongside an earlier body of work that had investigated the experiences of immigrant women of color who serve as domestic workers and paraprofessional nursing assistants and home care workers (Bakan and Stasiulis 1995; Carty 2003; Colen 1989, 1990, 1995; Foner 1994; Glenn 2010; Hondagneu Sotelo 2001; Parreñas 2001).

The literature on the migration of health professionals has investigated the role of nation states, transnational labor recruitment firms, educational and credentialing institutions, and other global actors who select, recruit, and train health care workers from abroad for work in health care institutions in advanced economies. The Philippines has garnered considerable attention as an empirical case study to document a particular case of labor migration where health care workers, specifically nurses, leave their homes educated and trained for the global labor market through sophisticated processes of education, labor recruitment, and government policy (Brush and Sochalski 2007; Choy 2003; Guevarra 2010; Rodriguez 2010; Ortiga 2014).

Unlike the organized and systematic education, transnational recruitment, and labor brokering processes that create a steady pipeline of nurses from nursing schools in the Philippines and India, for example, to hospitals and nursing homes in the United States (Banerjee 2022; George 2005; Guevarra 2010; Rodriguez 2010; Ortiga 2017, 2018; Walton-Roberts 2012, 2015), participants in this study became care workers—nurses, disability support professionals, and health care administrators—while in the United States. These men and women arrived in the United States through established migration channels made possible by U.S. immigration policies.

Bringing insights from U.S. immigration scholarship to bear, this book draws attention to the role of formal and informal social networks formed by West Africans as well as their entrepreneurial initiatives around the provision of care. This study thus highlights meso-level actors that tap into a reservoir of immigrant labor to create health care workers in destination countries. This book's intent in doing so is to shed light on this army of caregivers who are on the front lines of care and who are invisible in the eyes of mainstream and in the scholarship focused on the global recruitment of a professional health care labor force.

Migrants Who Care adds to our understanding of the U.S. health care industry and the lived experiences of immigrant workers by shedding light on the experiences of previously middle-class West African immigrants who care for adult/older adult populations upon migration and face downward or ambiguous social or occupational mobility because of their entry into care occupations. This was the case for Albert, whom we met earlier in this chapter. He was an economist and university lecturer in Sierra Leone prior to migration and held a master's degree. After migrating to the United States, he first sought employment in the field of economic policy. He even described an attempt to gain employment at the main offices of the World Bank, where, after making the shortlist of finalists for a policy analyst position, his application was turned down. After many attempts to gain employment with credentials earned from Sierra Leone, he got increasingly frustrated and desperate. Recognizing his desperation, a friend of his who is also an immigrant from Sierra Leone told him to seek employment in a group home. In the application process, the friend advised Albert to take his master's degree off his résumé so that he would not seem overqualified.

This book invests in an understanding of the lives and experiences of African immigrants like Albert, caring for a diverse group of care recipients, including African Americans and lower-income disabled patients who rely on state-funded Medicaid programs. Upon entering the care industry, especially in certain devalued niches, these immigrants encounter racialization and racism in U.S. society as well as downward occupational and social mobility. Because most of the research participants came from societies where long-term care of the elderly or people with disabilities was undertaken by family members or hired help in the home, they had to acclimatize to the care for vulnerable older adults and disabled individuals in institutional settings. Through this focus on a group of immigrant workers, most of whom were not paid care workers prior to migration, I ask the question: How do immigrant workers "learn to care?" In answering this question, I focus on the transformational processes that study participants undergo as they become paid care workers in the United States. By investigating the experiences of university-educated and previously middle-class immigrants and their strategies for coping with the class inconsistencies and incongruences arising from their entry into this field of work, I also extend the focus on gender and race central to this point to the literature on migrant health and domestic care workers. I highlight how class status prior to migration shapes the identities of Black immigrant care workers. *Migrants Who Care* also highlights West African immigrants' role as labor brokers who tap into their local ethnic and immigrant communities to channel coethnics into this much-needed global labor market.

THEORETICAL ANCHORS AND RECENT INNOVATIONS IN CONCEPTUALIZING CARE WORK

Conceptual formulations in care work seek to develop an integrated framework to understand skilled and semi-skilled work in home and institutional health care settings and paid reproductive labor in the home. For example, sociologists Mary Zimmerman, Jacqueline Litt, and Christine Bose define care work as "the multifaceted labor that produces the daily living conditions that make basic human health and well-being possible" (Zimmerman, Litt, and Bose 2006, 4). Their conceptualization of care work includes domestic tasks such as housekeeping and food production, as well as tasks such as "nursing the sick, looking after and nursing children, and assisting the disabled and elderly" (Zimmerman et al. 2006, 4). Sociologist Rhacel Parreñas notes that the activities of daily living that most care workers perform are essential and enhance the recipient's productivity. Also conceptualizing care work as physical activities that enhance the daily productive capabilities of others, sociologist Paula England and her co-authors note, "the care provider enhances the recipient's human capabilities (e.g., physical, emotional, and cognitive skills and proclivities of empathy and self-discipline" (England, Budig, and Folbre 2002, 455). They also consider the emotional and cognitive dimensions of the labor performed by care workers. Other works similarly highlight the emotional and affective nature of the labor care workers perform (Boris and Parreñas 2010; Diamond 1992; Dodson and Zincavage 2007; Duffy et al. 2015; Gottfried and Chun 2018; Stacey 2011). Sociologists Heide Gottfried and Jennifer Jihye Chun emphasize that care work enhances recipients' human capabilities, noting that as a form of "intimate labor," care work "produces affective relations, nurturance, healing, that enhance worker's capacities to labor and release labor's productive capabilities. Care creates something novel, generating affective relations, forms of life, and well-being" (Gottfried and Chun 2018: 5). The relational and emotional demands of work, or what sociologist Arlie Hochschild (1983) terms "emotional labor," sometimes compels workers to match their feelings and visible self-presentations to organizational or managerial requirements (Leidner 1993; Lopez 2006; Stacey 2011; Rodriquez 2014).

Scholars have debated aspects of emotional labor, for example, the aspect of organizational "social engineering" (Lopez 2006) or the extent to which employers have the power to control workers' emotions (Erickson and Stacey 2013; Leidner 1993; Lopez 2006; Rodriquez 2014). Studies have shown that emotional labor can have negative consequences, as it requires a "transmutation" of private feelings to public displays of emotion, which can then lead to workers' alienation from their own feelings (Lopez 2006; Rodriquez 2014; Stacey 2011). Building on this, other care work scholars have maintained that, while aspects of the work, for example, the personal care performed by nursing assistants, can be demanding and often unpleasant, the close encounters fostered through care can engender genuine feelings of closeness and intimacy. Thus, care work can engender both alienation and "empowering forms of emotional labor" (Stacey 2011, 10).

Interrogating the emotional and affective consequences of work that involves close and intimate ties between caregiver and care recipient, a strand of care work scholarship has highlighted the intrinsic rewards of care. Drawing mostly from the experiences of low-wage, low-prestige, home/elder care workers, these scholars have argued that care workers gain a lot of intrinsic rewards (job satisfaction, love, affect, and other positive emotions) in the absence of extrinsic rewards (adequate wages, attractive benefits, and so on). This body of work has posited intrinsic and extrinsic rewards of care as dichotomous and conflicting, with intrinsic rewards serving as compensation for the lack of extrinsic rewards (Coe 2019; Dwyer 2013; England 2005; Folbre et al. 2012; Folbre 2012; Rodriquez 2014; Stacey 2005, 2011). Yet, as the ensuing chapters will show, for many Black African immigrants to the United States, entry-level care jobs do provide extrinsic rewards for immigrant workers. These include a point of entry into the labor market, a livelihood, and, for many, the opportunity to send remittances home and a pathway to more professional segments in health care. While they encountered difficulties when they first became care workers, and challenges within institutional care settings, this book will show how West African immigrants also gain tremendous intrinsic rewards and develop prosocial motivations (the desire to help others) (Folbre et al. 2012) after being immersed in their jobs.

More recently, sociologist Cynthia Cranford has added a useful intersectional dimension to the discussion of emotions in care work, by exploring emotional labor within the context of the "complex power dynamic between recipients and workers who encounter different axes of oppression" (Cranford 2020, 11). Cranford focuses on the emotional labor performed by low-wage personal care assistants, often immigrant women of color, who care for recipients with various disabilities. By highlighting the relational aspect of care and bringing in much-needed perspectives from disability studies, Cranford investigates not only how able-bodied workers manage their own emotions but also how disabled care recipients who receive state-subsidized care manage theirs. This book builds on this scholarship on emotional labor. By focusing on care work as it takes place in institutional settings or home settings as mediated through ethnic labor markets, I explore how institutional structures and ethnic resources help or hinder care workers' emotional labor. I pay attention to West African immigrants' subjective understanding of their caregiving roles and under what conditions they develop genuine feelings of affection and intimate care relations with their care recipients. Like sociologist Clare Stacey (2011), I argue that the context of the work can shape employer's emotional labor; that is, whether they experience their emotions as alienating and constrained or pleasurable and rewarding. Like sociologist Cynthia Cranford (2020), by studying able-bodied, highly educated, previously middle-class Black immigrants who care for a diverse group of care recipients, including poor, disabled, African Americans relying on state-subsidized care, I am interested in how emotional labor is deployed and experienced by workers and care recipients positioned across various axes of oppression. Unlike Cranford, I focus on only one aspect of the relational dyad; that is, the experience of workers.

BLACK IMMIGRANTS' EXPERIENCES OF RACE, ETHNICITY, AND LABOR IN THE UNITED STATES

Through a deep investment in excavating the experiences of Black African immigrants, *Migrants Who Care* adds to our understanding of U.S. immigration. Existing sociological research that has looked at Black immigrants in the U.S. labor force has focused largely on Black/white interactions or on race relations among native-born and foreign-born Blacks in white-dominated and controlled work environments and contexts (Kasinitz and Vickerman 2001; Vickerman 1999, 2001; Waters 1990 2001). Reflecting patterns in Black immigration before 1980, this literature has generally focused on Caribbean Black immigrants residing in New York City (Foner 1987; Kasinitz and Vickerman 2001) and has extrapolated from findings specific to this group to make universal claims about Black immigrant identity (Waters 1990 2001; Vickerman 2001). The existing discussion of Black immigrants has largely centered around debates of whether culture and socialization (socialization in majority-Black premigration contexts, hardworking ethos, and immigrant orientations), or structure (racism and immigrant selectivity) account for disparities in achievement and labor market experiences between U.S.-born Blacks and immigrant Blacks (Hamilton 2019; Imoagene 2017; Model 2008; Medford 2019; Patterson 2006). A related and contested assertion in this literature is that first-generation Black immigrants in the United States gain upward mobility and success by stressing their ethnic particularities and through distancing themselves from the associated racism and negative associations with African Americans (Habecker 2012; Jackson 2010; Waters 1990, 2001; Vickerman 1999). Some studies highlight the role of employer preference for immigrant Blacks over African Americans in incentivizing this distancing (Vickerman 1999, 2007; Waters 2001).

Comparatively lesser effort has been expended in investigating race relations and identities in contexts where Blacks (foreign-born or native-born) predomi-

nate or in settings where a racially and culturally diverse workforce predomi-
nates. This book questions the assertion that ethnicity is a positive shield for all
Black immigrants, puts the assertion that employers prefer foreign-born Blacks
to native-born Blacks to the test, and shifts the existing emphasis on the Black/
white racial binary through its focus on the health care industry that has long
attracted a racially and ethnically diverse native-born and immigrant labor force
(Batalova 2020; Boris and Klein 2012; Hine 1989; Choy 2003; George 2005;
Glenn 2010; Wingfield 2019; Kingma 2005; Yeates 2009). I nuance our understanding of race and ethnicity among Black immigrants in the United States by
casting a qualitative lens on African immigrants' experiences and racial encounters within and across three broad health care work settings: (1) worksites where
African immigrants form the majority of employees (such as African-owned
home health care agencies or day centers for adults with intellectual disabilities);
(2) work settings where immigrants, especially immigrants from the global south,
are significantly represented in certain specializations and segments (e.g., elder
care); and (3) workplaces where white workers make up the majority (e.g., oncology units of prestigious hospitals). By investigating African immigrant experiences in diverse and varied work settings, I examine how the following factors
shape Black immigrant identities and experiences: the particularities of specific
occupations; the social organization of workplaces, including the racial/ethnic,
national, and gender composition of the workforce; and specific work contexts
and relations. Through the analysis of race, class, gender, and ethnicity among
recent African immigrants, I also interject an intersectional lens into the discussions of contemporary immigration in the United States.

STUDYING AFRICAN IMMIGRANT HEALTH CARE WORKERS

Migrants Who Care is based on interviews and ethnographic research conducted
at the offices of eight privately owned home care and disability support agencies
in Metropolitan Washington, DC, between 2010 and 2015. The agencies were
owned and operated by African immigrants from five nations sampled for this
study (Ghana, Nigeria, Sierra Leone, Liberia, and Cameroon)[10] and hired predominantly West African staff, whom they placed in private home care settings.
The workers they hired were mainly direct support professionals (DSP)—home
health aides (HHA) and other paraprofessional staff—but they also hired professional nurses. I chose home care and disability support businesses that were
owned and operated by West Africans as work sites to conduct field observation
rather than other institutional settings, like hospitals or nursing homes, to systematically map out and trace the processes that have facilitated the clustering of West
Africans in health care and to investigate their dual role as laborers and entrepre-
neurs/labor brokers responsible for channeling coethnics into health care work.

I focused attention on one of the most successful African-owned health care companies in that area that provided care for adults with intellectual disabilities, consisting of day programming and round-the-clock care in residential (group) homes. This company, which I call Worldwide, was founded by an immigrant couple from Sierra Leone, West Africa, and run by their second-generation (U.S.-born) adult children. Most individuals for whom they cared were older African Americans adults. All the care recipients exhibited various forms of intellectual disabilities, ranging from mild to severe. Some also had severe physical disabilities, diagnoses of mental illness, and other medical problems. Sierra Leone was the dominant nationality among the staff. The company also employed a minority of native-born American staff, most of whom were African American. Most of the staff were paraprofessional DSPs, but they also hired professionals, namely, qualified intellectual disability professionals (QIDPs), house managers, licensed practical nurses (LPNs), and registered nurses (RNs).

I conducted semi-structured, in-depth qualitative interviews with sixty-six West African immigrant health care workers (nurse practitioners, registered and licensed practical nurses, DSPs, and owners/managers of heath care businesses). They worked within various occupational settings in the health and long-term care industry (hospitals, nursing homes, group homes like the ones operated by Worldwide, and private homes) and cared for a diverse group of care recipients. Clients included vulnerable older adults in suburban nursing homes who tended to be mostly white; a younger, mostly African American population in city hospitals, private homes, and residential group homes; and a more racially diverse population in suburban hospitals.

Fifty-four interview subjects were women and twelve were men. Interviewees ranged in age from early twenties to late sixties. The interviews were conducted in the summer months (May–August) between 2010 and 2012. Care worker interviews covered questions about motivations and experiences of migration; work histories; pathways into and experiences in care work; relations with clients, co-workers, and supervisors; job satisfaction and difficulties; and future job prospects. For the owners and administrators of health care businesses, I asked open-ended questions regarding background and education in health care and/or health care administration; qualifications in the field; and descriptions of daily work experiences. I also asked questions relating to their clients' demographics; funding; training, disciplining, and recruitment of nursing and home health care and disability support staff; the ethnic and national makeup of staff; and their assessments of African nurses and disability support professionals.

In the summer of 2015, I returned to the field and conducted additional ethnographic work at the day program at Worldwide and more interviews with their staff, including a few follow-up interviews. In the intervening time, having moved to Connecticut in 2013, I have pursued informal interactions with the primarily Ghanaian immigrant community in the Hartford area who are also heavily involved in health care (primarily home care). These informal interactions and conversations also inform this book. I provide further details about methodological choices, the work settings and contexts, occupational groups, and the research sample in the methodological appendix.

ORGANIZATION OF THE BOOK

Chapter 1, "Moving to America," provides the conditions and context for understanding contemporary African immigration. This chapter draws from compelling individual narratives to chart the processes that cause Africans to leave their homelands. It explores the political economy in the nation states in West Africa, including the impact of neoliberal structural adjustment policies, as well as sociopolitical issues such as political unrest, wars/conflict, and gender inequality that serve as push factors for this group. It also discusses the modes and channels through which African immigrants enter and settle in the United States, focusing on family reunification, diversity, refugee, and employment provisions in the U.S. immigration regime. It analyzes the functions and effects of U.S. immigration policies on the lives, experiences, and labor force trajectories of contemporary immigrants, showing how these policies result in the erasure of premigration human capital while simultaneously providing legalized pathways to enter the primary labor market. This chapter concludes that access to legal immigration status and the specific terms of their entry into the US position West Africans to enter formal and institutional health care work.

Chapter 2, "Pathways and Entryways into Care," situates West African immigrants in the United States, focusing on their work lives. Building on sociologist Clare Stacey's concept of "caring trajectories," this chapter traces participants' entry into care work and highlights how they become concentrated in this line of work. It shows how these immigrants navigate settlement in the United States while dealing with problems such as the downgrading of their educational credentials earned from home, racial discrimination, and blocked opportunities in other sectors of the U.S. labor market. Presenting the lived experiences of individual immigrants, this chapter argues that racialized demands in the health care industry, as well as the agency of individual men and women, combine to facilitate the entry of this immigrant group into the health care field. It demonstrates how West African immigrants activate social and ethnic networks in the face of discrimination, creating a distinct and vibrant health care labor niche.

Chapter 3, "The Business of Care: Ethnic Entrepreneurship in Care," extends the focus on how ethnic networks create the West African health care labor supply, by showing how West Africans have formed businesses that capitalize on the labor of their coethnics and a racialized market for care. These businesses, embedded within immigrant social networks, cater to some of the most underserved populations. In ethnographic detail, this chapter provides the origin story of three select ethnic businesses and the personal narratives of these workers/ entrepreneurs. It highlights the role West African immigrants play as labor brokers and employers who produce, repackage, and deploy immigrants as workers whose labor conforms to ethical, regulatory, disciplinary, and bureaucratic norms in the DC care work landscape. It investigates how these entrepreneurs view their role and service both to the workers they hire and the recipients of care, and the challenges they face in navigating the Washington, DC, health care bureaucracy. In sum, this chapter provides empirical support for one of the central arguments of the book: that the social capital created in immigrant ethnic networks and businesses perpetuate and fuel West African immigrant labor streams into the health care industry.

Chapter 4, "Disability Support: The Transformation of Immigrants into Care Workers," takes the reader more closely into Worldwide, one of the businesses in the study, and sheds light on the people who receive care. Worldwide operates a day program for adults with intellectual disabilities. Through the lens of disability support, this chapter explores a key gendered dynamic: how immigrant men and women from non-health care backgrounds cope with their entry into care work in similar but also different ways. At this point in the book, I develop the concept of "class ambivalence" to trace the contradictory class location of middleclass African men and women who face downward social and occupational mobility because of certain tasks associated with care work but simultaneously earn higher incomes than they did back home while working in environments controlled by coethnics. I focus on the subjective identities and systems of meaningmaking that they develop and the transformations that happen as participants become produced, repackaged, and deployed as care workers. This chapter highlights the emotional labor of disability support, as well as the feelings of affection, engendered through the intimate relations in care work. By the conclusion of chapter 4, the repackaging of immigrants into health care workers is complete. I show how West African immigrants who were reluctant to become care workers remain in the field, citing the non-pecuniary and intrinsic rewards that come from working with adults with physical and intellectual disabilities.

Chapter 5, "Patient-Provider Interactions and Professional Identities in Nursing," continues the themes of meaning making and the development of subjective identities but shifts focus to highlight West African immigrants' labor in the professional ranks of the heath care occupational hierarchy. Chapter 5 centers around their professional experiences in bedside nursing. Here, I highlight nurse-patient interactions with a focus on how race and ethnicity intersect to shape the experiences of African immigrants. This chapter illuminates their experiences of racial discrimination. It highlights a specific form of racial animus toward Africans that I conceptualize as "African-origin discrimination." This chapter also examines strategies for survival and upward mobility within the context of racialized hierarchies in the nursing field. In this chapter, I extend the book's central argument on racial and gendered inequalities, this time by looking at racism and workplace discrimination that West African immigrants encounter upon entering the professional ranks of the health care industry. I articulate the concept of "professional distancing," which refers to a rhetorical move employed by some nurses to distance themselves from coethnics in specific work contexts as a strategy for upward mobility. I offer this concept as an addition to our knowledge of the complicated intersections of race and ethnicity in the experiences of Black African immigrants in the United States.

Chapter 6, "Nursing a Pathway to the American Dream," brings the discussion of work in separate segments (nursing, disability support, home care) together. Taking a holistic view of West Africans in the health care industry, this chapter discusses the rewards of work: extrinsic, (such as remuneration, material success, upward social mobility) and the intrinsic and prosocial (such as job satisfaction, community, and transnational health advocacy), versus the costs of work (hostile work environments, class ambivalence, racism, over work and burnout, and physical strain). This chapter poses the question: "Is health care (especially nursing) a pathway to the American dream?" To address this question, I venture beyond the work lives and highlight aspects of the personal lives, communities, and transnational ties that study participants form. I investigate whether the labor concentration in health care extends to the African immigrant 1.5 and second generations (immigrants who migrated as children and the children of African immigrants) using the concept of the "immigrant bargain" (Louie 2012; Smith 2006; Suárez Orozco and Suárez Orozco, 1995).

The conclusion of the manuscript returns to the major findings and themes of the book. I highlight how West Africans have come to create an occupational niche in health care provision; reiterate their contributions to the health care industry in the United States; and show how this study on West African immigrants extends the literature on migrant health care workers to encompass the production, repackaging, and deployment of immigrants with non-health care backgrounds into care workers upon migration. In the conclusion, I revisit how *Migrants Who Care* contributes to the scholarship on race and U.S. immigration. I end with policy implications of this work, especially as they relate to the current crises of aging and care in the United States and the global coronavirus pandemic.

1 · MOVING TO AMERICA

We saw this ad in the newspaper which told us that we could get a green card if we came over here. Like the visa lottery. So, we put that in [we applied], so surprisingly we won the lottery. It was a decision to either stay where we were ... cause we were in South Africa at that time with a contract, because my husband is a physician. But we looked at it. Over there we were getting [a] work permit every year, and then here comes this lottery that tells us that we'll get the green card and then become a citizen here.

—Kate, RN, Ghana

I came to the United States to join my fiancée, and then later, wife. She is an African American. We met in Tokyo while I was doing my master's program. She came to Tokyo to complete an exchange program. So, I joined her in 2000. Unfortunately, it [the relationship] did not work out.

—Albert, QIDP, Sierra Leone

I used to live in Kono district [Sierra Leone] during the war when the rebels invaded the district in 1992, we came to Freetown [capital city]. We were there for a year, and things were not changing so.... and life was so hard, and I am the bread winner for the family, so I just decided to move to the U.S. Fortunately, I was able to get a visitor's visa.

—Fatima, RN, Sierra Leone

These words capture the motivations for migration for West African immigrants, and the various modes of migration through which they come. Like Kate, Albert, and Fatima, all the immigrants I encountered entered the country through legal channels, with some entering on a permanent basis (mostly as family reunification immigrants, diversity visa lottery winners, or as refugees). Others who entered on a temporary basis, for example as students or on tourist visas, had been able to change their status and become lawful permanent residents, and later naturalized U.S. citizens. Most, like Albert, did so through marriage to U.S. citizens, while others benefited from employment-based preferences in immigration law. Their legal status explains to a large degree how members of this regional immigrant group have been able to establish themselves as part of a heavily regulated, bureaucratic labor force in an occupational category (health care) with stringent credentialing requirements and law enforcement safeguards.[1]

To frame this book's discussion of paid care work performed by West African immigrants in the United States, this chapter addresses the following questions: What makes a person motivated and able to come to the United States? How do they come, and is there a relationship between how one enters the United States and the type of work one is later able to do? As sociologist and demographer Tod Hamilton has noted, understanding immigrant incorporation into a receiving society requires gaining an understanding of the process through which they were selected to leave their home countries and the pathways through which they come (2019). This chapter takes on this charge and paints a picture of contemporary African immigration to the United States. Much like the participants in sociologists Susan Pearce, Elizabeth Clifford, and Reena Tandon's (2011) sweeping study of immigrant women in the United States, those I interviewed identified various and complex motivations for migration and traversed various immigration categories and statuses during their tenure in the United States. They also took varied pathways into paid care work after migration and experienced different mobility tracks within health care occupations, due to age/life stage at time of migration, class background, lack of opportunity in other sectors of the U.S. labor market, and access to social capital through family and immigrant social networks.

Contrary to the realities of other immigrant groups that have gained a lot of popular and some scholarly attention—such as recipients of the Deferred Action for Childhood Arrivals program[2]—who claim symbolic and cultural membership in American society but face legal barriers to full incorporation into the United States (Enriquez 2020, 2017a, 2017b; Gonzales 2016; Patler 2018), study participants have been able to enter the U.S. health care bureaucracy without many legal barriers. While almost all of them started at the bottom of the professional hierarchies of the health care field, their location in health care occupations represents relative advantage in the labor market. Relative to other employment niches populated by unauthorized immigrants—such as domestic work in private households (Carty 2003; Chang 2000; Colen 1989; Francisco-Menchavez 2018; Hondagneu-Sotelo 2001; Parreñas 2001), the day labor workforce (Purser 2009), informal landscaping (Ramirez and Hondagneu-Sotelo 2009), agriculture (Holmes 2013; Rothenberg 2000), and street vending (Estrada 2019; Estrada and Hondagneu-Sotelo 2013; Rosales 2020)—that operate in the shadows, are unregulated, precarious, and exploitative, the health care field is generally heavily regulated and supervised. As this book will show, legal immigration status, (access to permanent residency status and naturalized citizenship) has allowed some West African immigrants to enter health care and, in some instances, to gain upward mobility across segments in the health care industry.

In the next section of this chapter, I will show the motivations for migration for individual research participants and the structural conditions at home that compelled them to leave. Following that, I will investigate specific immigration policies and how they have affected study participants' experiences. These policies dictate whether and how people can migrate and, once in the receiving country, their options for employment, their legalized tenures, and their pathways to citizenship. In discussing these policies, I trace their impact on individual study participants' immigration and labor market outcomes. In this, I follow a line of scholarship that has argued that the U.S. immigration regime, including its visa provisions and stipulations, segment immigrant workers in the labor market in ways not necessarily tied to their skills, abilities, or preferences (Gowayed 2022; Hagan, Hernández-León, and Demonsant 2015).

MOTIVATIONS FOR AND MODES OF MIGRATION

West African research participants left their homes for multiple reasons and made their way to the United States using various immigration pathways and often through circuitous journeys. Yenoh Sesay, for example, had received a government scholarship in Sierra Leone in the 1970s that had allowed her to pursue further education in what was then the Soviet Union. She then returned to Sierra Leone and became a finance officer in a governmental agency dedicated to exporting and marketing agricultural produce. By her own description, Yenoh led a comfortable existence. She first came to the United States temporarily, to visit her niece. Yenoh was one of a few participants who indicated an initial reluctance to come to the United States: "I have travelled to a lot of countries and [my niece] wanted me to come to America. You know at first, I resisted, because of all the propaganda . . . you know shootings, killings. . . . these things that we heard back home that America is a very dangerous place. . . . So, it took me a long time to make up my mind to come."

Yenoh arrived in 1992 on a tourist or visitor visa, after her niece allayed her fears about gun violence in Virginia where she lived. She brought her eleven-month-old daughter but left her older son back home. While on the visit, she received news that her agency was closing, thus rendering her unemployed. The civil war in Sierra Leone that had begun the year before was intensifying, and relatives and friends urged her to remain. She was very reluctant, not least because she had left her son in the care of relatives. As she said: "So, they [family members at home] said we'll take care of your son. You know he'll be in good hands. We'll take care of him. So, don't think of coming back home. And so, it was a bitter pill to swallow. And then my family here too [in the United States] they were convincing me not to go back.

And so finally after getting numerous telephone calls and letters from my brothers and sisters [from] back home ... I decided to stay. And that's when I started the process of, you know, getting my papers straightened out."

Yenoh filed a petition for asylum and, after a lengthy legal process, earned the ability to stay. In the system of differentiated grades of access to citizenship and full membership in U.S. society (Parreñas 2001) engendered by U.S. immigration policy, she successfully converted from a temporary status to permanent legal residence. She emphasized that, had family members not pushed her so hard to stay in the United States, she would have returned to Sierra Leone. Working as a registered nurse with a master's degree when we met, she found she was unable to find work in her field of financial management after she decided to settle in the United States.

Yenoh's story shows the disjuncture between conceptual and policy categories and the lived experiences of immigrants. Economic considerations played as significant a role in her decision to stay in the United States as political instability, but only the latter supported her classification as an asylum-seeker. Like many immigrants to the United States, Yenoh's experience transgresses and blurs the dichotomous lines drawn in the immigration literature (and in the prevailing international regime governing refugees) between economic migrants and political refugees. Thus, her example and the examples of many others reinforce the need for global migration scholars and policymakers to avoid "categorical fetishism" (Crawley and Skeplaris 2018) in addressing the needs and realities of migrants and refugees.

Rebekah Sankoh, who also became a registered nurse while in the United States, also arrived on a visitor's visa from Sierra Leone, but unlike Yenoh, she came specifically due to economic reasons. Prior to migration in the early nineties, Rebekah was a public school teacher. At that time, public sector employees in Sierra Leone were generally poorly paid and went without pay for months at a time, as the government was crippled by corruption, economic crises, and budgetary failures (Conteh-Morgan and Dixon-Fyle 1999). The embrace of the austerity measures dictated by the Structural Adjustment Policies (SAP) advocated by the International Monetary Fund in Sierra Leone as well as other developing countries involved the curtailing of public expenditure, resulting in layoffs of public employees and the reduction of social services and safety nets for the most marginal of members in society (Adepoju 2000, 2001, 2002; Arthur 2009; Chang 2000). Several scholars have pointed to the particularly gendered nature and impact of the SAPs and have argued that women like Rebekah and their children have been disproportionately affected (Chang 2000; McFadden 1997; Sassen 1991). A single parent, Rebekah obtained a visitor's visa and made her way to the United States, leaving her daughter, then a toddler, behind. West African immigrants like Rebekah are, therefore, part of what historian Paul Zeleza (2009) has termed a "structural adjustment diaspora." They are businesspeople, professionals, and ordinary citizens who are forced to leave due to the worsening economic and social conditions in their countries of origin. Rebekah later adjusted her status to permanent residence through marriage to a U.S citizen, and her daughter joined her at the age of nine. At the time of our interview, she was a registered nurse and owned a home care and nurse staffing agency. Her daughter worked for the agency as a registered nurse.

While Yenoh and Rebekah had moved independently, other migrants, like Henricia Gottfried, from Ghana, had migrated to the United States to accompany or join their spouses. Henricia arrived with her husband, who had come to pursue graduate studies in a Washington, DC, area university in the early 1970s as part of the post-independence wave of contemporary African immigrants who had migrated, mostly to pursue further education in the United States (Arthur 2000; Donkor 2017). Both expected to return to Ghana after he completed his studies. However, while in the United Sates, the democratically elected government of Ghana was overthrown in a coup d'état led by Flight Lieutenant Jerry Rawlings, who later became the president of Ghana.[3] This coup ushered in a turbulent period characterized by political violence, disappearances, killings, and severe economic decline. This period also saw a related exodus of Ghanaian citizens (Donkor 2017). Under Rawlings's watch in the 1980s, Ghana implemented one of Africa's most stringent SAPs, which created economic and political turmoil (Donkor 2017). Henricia and her husband, therefore, decided to stay in the United States and forego their plans of returning to Ghana. Henricia, who had been a nurse and certified midwife in Ghana, learned she could not find work in health care because she held temporary legal status as a dependent on her husband's student visa. She had to work informally as a nanny to support her husband, who was studying for a graduate degree, and their three young children they had left in Ghana.

Henricia's case emphasizes that visa categories through which immigrants gain admittance to the United States place structural limitations on what they can achieve once in U.S. society. This plays out in the sorting and ranking of immigrants as workers. Immigrants who enter legally but on a temporary basis (e.g., on student visas or, like Henricia, who came as dependents of primary migrants on student visas, or those who arrive on visitor visas), have legal restrictions to finding gainful employment (Banerjee 2022). Those who are unauthorized are typically restricted to the most difficult, dirty, and dangerous jobs (Chang 2000; Gonzales 2016; Hall, Greenman, and Yi 2019; Purser 2009). For immigrants like Henricia, who trained in health care before migration, policies guiding skilled health care worker credentialing and licensing created another barrier. In line with scholarship finding that immigration and labor policies are disciplining forces that serve to position low-wage immigrants, especially women of color, into precarious labor conditions through their granting of zero or partial citizenship rights (Banerjee 2018; Chang 2000; Gleeson and Griffith 2020),

Henricia could not immediately work as a nurse, although she had RN qualifications when she arrived and had many years of experience working as a nurse
specializing in midwifery in Ghana. Like other participants with credentials
earned from their home countries, Henricia found re-credentialing expensive
and difficult since it involved enrolling in U.S. university programs. Nurses like
Henricia were forced to find work as home health aides, certified nursing assistants, nannies, or in other service sector jobs, such as the fast food industry, to
earn money to pay for nursing school, taking a route of "deskilling" (Ball 2004;
Pratt 1999; Raghuram and Kofman, 2004; Yeates 2009) that geographer Geraldine Pratt (1999), writing about Filipinas in Vancouver, British Columbia, characterized as moving from "registered nurse to registered nanny." The assemblage
of labor restrictions, education and credentialing regimes, occupational gatekeeping strategies, and immigration policies faced by Henricia and others creates a racialized, cheapened, and devalued labor pool of laborers caring for
vulnerable older adults, children, the infirm, and the disabled (Colen 1989, 1995;
Chang 2000; McGregor 2007; Pratt 1999).

As the cases of Yenoh, Rebekah, and Henricia suggest, immigration policies
shape the trajectories of immigrants in the United States and have remarkable
power to help or hinder the prospects of immigrants who otherwise possess
human capital, talent, drive, and potential (Gonzales 2016; Gowayed 2022).

In the sections that follow, I describe the major developments in U.S. immigration policy that pertain to study participants, to show how these policies and
the visa categories embedded therein shape the immigration pathways and prospects of contemporary African immigrants in the United States

IMMIGRATION POLICIES AND STRUCTURAL FACTORS
IN DETERMINING MIGRATION JOURNEYS

When he married a U.S. citizen, Albert Kamara, whose words appear at the
opening of this chapter, benefited from family reunification provisions enshrined
in the 1965 Immigration and Nationality Act, also known as the Hart-Celler
Immigration Act. The 1965 Immigration Act overturned the explicit racial under-
pinnings of U.S. immigration law enshrined in the 1924 Immigration Act, by
doing away with numeric quotas that favored Western European countries. Historians have credited the 1965 Act with diversifying the U.S. population, as it
opened large-scale immigration from Latin America, Asia, the Caribbean, and,
to a lesser extent, Africa, and the Middle East—regions that had been underrepresented in prior eras (Hamilton 2019; Jimenez 2017; Kibria et al. 2014; Portes
and Rumbaut 2014). The 1965 Immigration Act also made family relationships
with U.S. citizens or permanent residents a major preference category for admission to the United States (Portes and Rumbaut 2014; Pearce et al. 2011). As a result,
67 percent of legal immigrants to the United States enter under this provision in

immigration law, when adult U.S. citizens petition for their immediate relatives (spouses, minor children, parents, and, to a lesser extent, siblings) to join them from abroad or to adjust their status within the United States (Hooper and Salant 2018). Although many family petition categories exist, the least complicated pathway to permanent residence is when U.S. citizens petition for immediate family members—spouses, parents, and unmarried children under twenty-one years of age, as these family members are not subject to annual visa limits. These petitions for permanent residency take, on average, six months, and the recipients become permanent residents immediately (Enriquez 2020). Petitions for adult children over twenty-one years and their spouses, and other extended family members, such as adult siblings, have considerable wait times, sometimes one to two decades, depending on national origin (Banerjee 2022; Enriquez 2020). Sophie Margai, a former athletic coach from Sierra Leone, and her family illustrate the sometimes-convoluted workings of family reunification: Sophie's sister became a U.S. citizen through marriage to a U.S. citizen she had met while living in Sierra Leone. After moving to the United States and becoming a naturalized citizen, Sophie's sister then sponsored Sophie's mother, and Sophie's mother subsequently sponsored Sophie. Although the wait time for processing was long, armed with a green card upon arrival and living with and aided financially by her mother and sister, Sophie was quickly able to enter nursing school.

Albert Kamara, discussed earlier, had met and married his African American fiancée while they were both students in Japan and described their partnership in romantic terms. His marriage allowed him to move to the United States and gain permanent residence status, although, as he told, me, "unfortunately it [the relationship] did not work out." Unlike Albert, most of the research subjects, male and female, who had arrived on temporary visas (such as student or visitor visas) and legalized their status through marriage entered these marriages while in the United States. Their spouses were often coethnics who had become naturalized U.S. citizens. They were less than forthcoming about the details of those marriages, and many simply said, "I got my papers through marriage." The timing of these marriages and the connection to obtaining permanent legal status suggests to me that some were strategic marriages contracted for immigration reasons, or "marriage for papers" as widely understood in immigrant communities (Enriquez 2020). Though reluctant to provide details of how these marriages were contracted and if or under what circumstances they were dissolved, it is possible that such "marriages of convenience," as sociologist Heba Gowayed found in her study of Syrian refuges, may subject women in particular to increased vulnerability, exploitation, harassment, coercion, and sabotage from perpetrators with promises of "papers."

West Africans who entered the United States as refugees, or those like Yenoh, a nurse mentioned previously, who claim asylum from within the United States, benefit from relatively more recent legislation: the Refugee Act, which President

Jimmy Carter signed into law in 1980. This law brought U.S. refugee policy in line with international law and practice, dispensing with the earlier policy that favored refugees and asylum seekers fleeing communist regimes (Portes and Rumbaut 2014).[4] The increased numbers of African refugees entering the United States reflect this new focus of immigration policy and the cyclical political crises in many parts of Africa (Gordon 1998; Arthur 2000, 2009; Hamilton 2019; Takyi and Konadu-Agyemang 2006). The study participants who arrived as refugees or gained asylum in the United States were mostly from Sierra Leone or Liberia.[5] But as Yenoh's story suggests, African immigrants straddle the rigid boundaries between refugees, economic migrants, and family migrants. Some participants, like Kezia Weekes, a licensed practical nurse from Liberia, did not arrive as refugees but remained in the United States under temporary protected status (TPS).[6]

Fatima Kamara is one of the Sierra Leonean and Liberian immigrants affected by war. She was forced to flee from armed conflict in rural Sierra Leone to the country's capital, Freetown. Displaced from her hometown, she found it difficult to eke out a living in Freetown. She characterized herself as fortunate when, after a year in Freetown, she was able to obtain a visitor's visa to the United States. Fatima's migration exemplified a migration stream charted by sociologist Saskia Sassen (1991), where women migrants from the global south first move from rural to urban areas. This process incorporates them within the orbit of capitalist expansion through work in gendered occupations in manufacturing in export processing zones, in the service, sex, and tourism sectors of developing economies. This insertion into the global economy ultimately facilitates migration to developed economies (Brennan 2004; Kempadoo 1999; Safa 1995). Scholars focusing on Africa have identified other push factors that motivate such migrations, including economic depression in rural Africa due to lack of investment in agricultural systems, limited technological innovation, drought and crop failures, declining prices of agricultural product, and political mismanagement (Arthur 2009); food crises, adverse climatic conditions, fluctuations in the international market for primary products, and other economic/political factors (Adepoju 1991, 2002); and gender-based violence and discrimination (Osirim 2011, 2012). While Fatima emphasized conflict, these factors also play a role in driving African emigration. Like Albert and Rebekah, the former teacher described earlier, she ultimately gained permanent residency status through marriage to a U.S. citizen.

In contrast to settlement through marriage, Harriet Williams, a Sierra Leonean registered nurse, had settled in the United States due to employment-based provisions in immigration law. The Immigration and Nationality Act of 1952 established the HI visa category, a nonimmigrant visa for employers who needed to hire foreign workers on a temporary basis.[7] The Immigration Nursing Relief Act of 1989 established nursing as an occupational category for such visas. This move allowed health care institutions to petition for nonimmigrant visas for foreign workers, reflecting the cyclical shortage of nurses in the United States.

Under the terms of this visa, an employer can employ nurses from abroad if they pass the licensure exam, and the nurse in question then becomes eligible to apply for permanent residency status after five years of employment (Banerjee 2022; Chang 2000; Choy 2003, McCabe 2012). The H1A visa was officially phased out in 1995, but the Nursing Relief for Disadvantaged Areas Act of 1999 created the H1C visa to allow for recruitment of foreign nurses to work in medically underserved areas. The H1C visa operated in a manner similar to the H1A, allowing for permanent residency after five years, but was discontinued in 2009 (McCabe 2012). None of the eight nurses in the sample who had nursing credentials before coming to the United States were recruited from abroad. So those who, like Harriet, obtained H1A or H1C visas, did so after they completed their studies and passed their board exams once in the United States. The employers, health care institutions in the United States, were able to petition on their behalf, and by the time we spoke, all had obtained permanent residency status.

Harriet had trained in Sierra Leone but came on a visitor's visa and completed additional training before receiving an offer from a hospital interested in sponsoring her visa application. She said of her decision to come to the United States: "I realized that in Sierra Leone, getting into the nursing profession after having gone to school for three-four years and all of that, you are still not recognized the way you would want to be recognized. You know, in terms of your educational goals, in terms of the fact that you went to school, you are educated but what you get in terms of future salary and financial goals it wasn't like worth it." Harriet also recalled that she had been advised by a friend back home that her "career will pay off big time" if she were to move to the United States.

Casandra Johnson, another U.S.-trained nurse, had entered the United States later in the 2000s, between the H1A visa's expiration and the H1C visa's establishment (McCabe 2012), and she, like several others, gained citizenship through marriage to a U.S. citizen. Some nurses who had graduated a few years prior to the time data was collected for this study detailed experiences of heartbreak and frustration as they waited for approval of their H1C visas due to the backlog of processing by immigration services. The evolution in the H1 visa categories shows how immigration policies and administrative procedures respond to the changing needs of the U.S. labor market. They also show the salience of immigration policies in shaping the entry and labor market trajectories of immigrants to the United States.

The final visa category that affected study participants was the diversity visa. The 1990 Immigration Act instituted the diversity visa lottery, which provided immigrant visas to countries with low rates of immigration to the United States. The visas are distributed annually via a lottery system with the aim of correcting some of the inequalities built into the pre-1965 immigration regime. The DV lottery, as it became popularly known, aims to diversify the immigrant population in the United States by allotting immigrant visas to countries with low rates of immigration to the United States and countries historically limited from migration prior to 1965 (Konadu-Agyemang and Takyi 2006). The DV lottery and the 1980 Refugee Act were responsible for the exponential increase in the recent migration of Africans to the United States (Anderson 2015; Arthur 2009; Hamilton 2019).

These policies are not just words on paper; they have life-changing consequences for West African immigrants like Kate Yeboah, a Ghanaian-trained registered nurse. She had moved to South Africa with her husband, who was a medical doctor. They were required to renew their work permits every year in South Africa, which they found burdensome. They entered the DV lottery and won the opportunity to start a new life in the United States. While Kate described the decision to enter the DV lottery as a highly rational one based on a specific weighing of options and goals, for Lara Bello, a registered nurse with a master's degree, winning the DV lottery provided her with a lifeline. She had migrated to England with her children from Nigeria. Her husband, who was in the military in Nigeria, had been appointed to be the defense attaché for the Nigerian embassy in London. She had gone ahead with their children to settle in, and her husband was scheduled to join them. However, before Lara's husband arrived in Britain, there was a coup d'état in Nigeria. His appointment never materialized, and due to his involvement with the previous government, he could not leave Nigeria. Lara, meanwhile, could not return to Nigeria with her children due to the volatile political situation. Based on the advice of family members, she became a nurse in England to earn money to sustain herself and her children. Winning the DV lottery years later allowed her to make a new life for herself and her children in the United States, since she had become estranged, by then, from her husband. As she said, rather dramatically, about her choice to live and work away from her home: "I had no choice, it's either I work to have money to feed my children, or they would starve."

Other recipients of diversity visas characterized their decisions to migrate as products of opportunity, luck, or happenchance, stating that winning the lottery allowed them to migrate for "adventure" or the opportunity to "broaden their horizons." Daisy Obi was a DV lottery winner who had been a registered nurse in Nigeria. She attributed her decisions to her being a restless personality who always sought out change and new adventures. She explained that she had travelled to many other countries and lived in other parts of the world: "I like to go to new places, meet new people and see new things. Just know what the world is all about." She presented herself as having a thirst for learning about different peoples and cultures. Initially, she did not intend to stay in the United States because, as she said, "I had a good job by Nigerian standards. As a nurse I was earning a good salary as per my own standards." However, other Nigerians told her that life would be good in the United States and there were plenty of opportunities to make money. According to Daisy, people in her social circle in Nigeria said that anyone who hadn't been to America hadn't been anywhere." They saw America as a land of opportunity. Partly inspired by these narratives, Daisy tried the DV lottery three times and won on the third try. She then quit her nursing job and migrated to the United States. Even though she was a qualified nurse in Nigeria with specialties in midwifery and public health, she had to work, first, in a service job at McDonald's. As she said: "I worked at McDonald's, but that was terrible for me, because it was not fun. When I came back [home from work], my legs swell up. I was not happy about it. Oh my God. I told my sister, I complain, complain, complain, complain. When I come back, I'm so tired. I want to sleep the whole day."

Daisy then got a job as a home health aide, which she found less difficult and better paid than working in the fast-food industry. She spoke fondly of some of the clients she worked with as a home health aide while she waited to get her credentials transferred and evaluated so she could go back to nursing.

Author and immigrant rights activist Grace Chang stated: "The notion that immigrants can be treated as expendable commodities, to be used then expelled from the country or simply from any public concern, has guided immigration law and labor practice throughout US labor history" (Chang 2000, 93). Study participants represent some of the realities of this approach to immigration policy. Their lives were structured and ordered by the provisions in the U.S. immigration regime on the one hand but also the workings of global capitalism and the actions of the sending states in West Africa on the other. Historical processes and present conditions characterized by wars/political instability, economic disaster, and social problems in sending states factored into individual-level decisions to migrate. Their experiences in the United States were mediated by their "legal" immigrant status. The fact that they had access to legal immigration status contributed to the ability of all research subjects, even those without health care backgrounds, to enter health care occupations after migration.[8] However, most could enter only at the lower tiers of the industry. Educational and credentialing regimes, as well as institutional gatekeeping mechanisms, resulted in some previously qualified health care workers having to start their lives over, usually by pursuing additional training for health care credentials. Subsequent chapters will explore the experiences of these immigrants within the health care industry and the challenges they faced as they navigated structural barriers such as ghettoization in certain occupational segments.

2 · PATHWAYS AND ENTRYWAYS INTO CARE

On a hot day in July, I visited the home of Clarice Johnson, a Liberian immigrant nurse. I arrived at our predetermined time, but she was not home; her eighteen-year-old daughter told me Clarice had worked an extremely long shift and would be home soon. We chatted for a while as I waited. The young woman struck me as intellectually curious, if a little shy. Clarice later arrived with her younger daughter, and the two sisters started arguing while Clarice and I began discussing her experiences as a licensed practical nurse. She had to interrupt the interview a few times to tell her daughters to keep it down.

Clarice had a slight build, but she was extremely energetic and active. She was still full of energy despite having completed a twelve-hour shift. I sat in the living area while she went back and forth from there to the kitchen of the small apartment. By the time we completed our interview, she had given the younger daughter a snack, instructed her to start her homework, and started dinner. The teenager, bored of the argument perhaps, had started watching TV. Clarice invited me to stay for dinner, but I declined politely, saying I had a long drive ahead of me. She insisted on packing some food for me to take home. I followed her into the kitchen. Speaking in a hushed tone, she told me she was surprised her older daughter had talked to me while I waited, as she was usually antisocial. She confided that she was worried about her daughter, who was disaffected and not doing well in school. As we walked back into the living room, Clarice said more audibly that she had been trying to convince her daughter to get a job as a home health aide, and that she had even contacted one of the major recruiting agencies whose owners she knew personally to get her a job. Hearing this, her daughter said, rudely, that she did not want to be a home health aide. She continued that she was born in America and, therefore, did not wish to "clean people's asses." Clarice turned to me and, in a hurt tone, said, "She thinks she is too good to do the work that I did to provide for them."

This dramatic family incident represents the pervasiveness of health care work in the worlds and minds of West African immigrants in the Washington,

DC, metropolitan area. The daughter's reaction illustrates the stigma associated with some caring tasks. It also shows the divergent views between immigrants and their U.S.-born children of direct care work as a viable employment pathway. At the same time, the younger woman's resistance belied another reality I saw, which is that immigrant mothers wielded significant influence over their daughters' decisions around health care work.

This chapter will focus on respondents like Clarice—first-generation immigrants from Nigeria, Ghana, Sierra Leone, Liberia, and Cameroon who work as health care workers and as labor market brokers and entrepreneurs in health care. Using the experiences of individual workers, I will trace workers' journeys into caring occupations, what sociologist Clare Stacey (2011) has termed "caring trajectories." While Stacey's respondents, primarily native-born citizens from Ohio and California, generally had provided unpaid care for a family member, friend, or neighbor, which then led them to pursue employment in paid caregiving, the subjects of this book, first-generation immigrants from West Africa, did not have such histories. Stacey's respondents cited their "natural ability" to care as the primary factor allowing them to assume responsibility for child and elder care in their families and why they found themselves in paid care. Convictions about "natural" caregiving abilities, according to Stacey, obscure what is "in fact a lifetime of constrained choices" with respect to caregiving obligation" (2011, 21).

Most of the subjects of this book came from middle-class households in their home countries, where hired help typically managed some domestic tasks. Rather than experiencing a "lifetime of constrained choices," their caring trajectories were launched after pivotal disruptive moments or turning points in their lives. For many, these moments of disruption started when they arrived in the United States and faced limited options in the labor market. Others had faced professional or personal setbacks after living in the United States for some time, and many more were ushered into care work through the influence of people I term "care pioneers,"[1] members of their ethnic networks who already were settled in the United States and, often, were care workers themselves. Many participants had faced a combination of these scenarios, and almost all the research subjects had worked in other low-wage service employment—as nannies, dishwashers in restaurants, servers in fast-food restaurants, or security guards—before entering health care work. Thus, rather than framing their care roles as "natural," many West African immigrants articulated care as an assemblage of skill sets or attributes that they had to learn or acquire in their journeys in the United States.

ENTERING CARE WORK

I grouped the immigrant care workers with whom I interacted roughly into three categories based on age/life stage at the time of migration. The first group comprised members of the immigrant 1.5 generation (who migrated as young children or in their pre-teen years, often with or to reunite with parents who had migrated prior). Sarah Josiah, an immigrant nurse from Liberia, is a case in point. Sarah arrived in the United States as a teenager. At the time of our interview, she was a nurse practitioner, an achievement of which she was very proud. However, Sarah's caring trajectory started after she got pregnant while still in high school. Her father, previously a prominent government official in Liberia, and her mother, a successful businesswoman, had undergone substantial downward mobility after they fled the civil war in their country and arrived in the United States. Now working as a security guard and a certified nursing assistant, respectively, and struggling to make ends meet, her father and mother were not able to support her financially. She needed to provide for her newborn daughter herself, so she became a certified nursing assistant. After the birth of her child, and while still working as a CNA, she started taking part-time classes at a community college to become a licensed practical nurse. While becoming an LPN normally takes two years, Sarah took six years to complete the qualification, as she balanced working full time, taking classes on and off, and caring for her daughter. Balancing her work as an LPN and taking still further classes, she later became a registered nurse. Eventually, she would practice nursing at the highest levels, as a nurse practitioner. As she pointed out during our conversation, during her career in health care, Sarah had occupied all the rungs in the nursing ladder. While other care work scholars have portrayed home care and nursing assistant work as leading to dead ends (Buch 2018; Coe 2019; Donkor 2017; Diamond 1992; Rodriquez 2014; Stacey 2011), Sarah's case and many more that I will highlight in this book show how some West African immigrants have parlayed entry-level positions in the health care industry into more professional ones and into opportunities for entrepreneurship.

The second group were young adults at the time of migration. They migrated in their late teens and early twenties and often derived from elite or middle-class backgrounds. For these first two groups, I delineated class background from parental occupation and educational background. Some in the second group came to the United States to attend university. For the most part, their parents could fund their education and life in the United States, or they had networks of kin already present in the United States who could connect them with work and other resources. Most started college intending to become professionals, such as lawyers, doctors, or engineers. They, like others in the first group, became care workers after disruptive moments, or what I term "life interruptions," such as financial difficulty resulting from parents' losing jobs; failure to gain admittance to graduate programs of their choice; or, in the case of some of the women, unplanned pregnancies that halted their career plans and forced them to find alternative means of survival. For this group, entering care work entailed a recalibration of life expectations and new ways of understanding and framing their life experiences.

Nelson Sandy is a member of the second group. A qualified intellectual disability professional when we met, he had migrated from Sierra Leone to California to attend college. His father was a prominent politician in Sierra Leone. Nelson's parents helped pay his university tuition, and he lived with a cousin while working various part-time jobs to fund his living expenses. Starting his college career at a community college, he then transferred to one of the most highly ranked and prestigious public universities in the United States. He graduated with a degree in political science, then moved to New York City after graduation and started a master's program in history. He planned to pursue a doctorate degree and to move on to a career in academia. He encountered a life interruption, however, when, after a difficult academic year, he lost his graduate funding and had to drop out of school. Disillusioned and despondent that his professional goals had not materialized, he moved to the Washington, DC, area, where he had other family. These family members helped him get a job at a Sierra Leonean-owned company that provided residential homes for adults with intellectual disabilities. He started off providing hands-on care for adults with severe physical and intellectual disabilities, but by the time we spoke, he was a supervisor of disability support aides employed by the company.

Nelson's experiences are illustrative of the research participants whose caring trajectories were launched after other professional pursuits failed. His experiences also hint at another transformation identified by sociologists Robert Emerson and Melvin Pollner (1976). At first reluctant to enter care work and perceiving the work as "dirty work," as they stayed longer in the field and as they achieved positions with increased responsibility and more earnings, the work eventually transformed from being "dirty work" to becoming more rewarding.

Musu Fofana, also from Sierra Leone, had come to the United States for college, as well. Musu's father was a high-level civil servant in Sierra Leone and, like Nelson's parents, could afford to sponsor his child's education in the United States. Musu also began at community college and lived with a relative, in her case an aunt in Ohio. She also transferred to a four-year state university, but her life interruption came before graduation. Her father ran into financial difficulties and could not afford to continue to pay for her education. Forced to drop out of university, she worked as a server in a fast food restaurant, as an assistant in a dry-cleaning facility, as a nanny, and doing data entry work in a large public hospital. She then joined the same Sierra Leonean-owned company as Nelson. Her mother knew the owner of the company before the latter migrated—a connection that helped Musu get the job. Musu started out as a DSP, providing hands-on care, and at the time of our meeting, she was a house manager supervising a residential household of individuals with various disabilities and the home care workers who cared for them.

The third group comprised immigrants who were in their mid-twenties to late fifties at the time of migration. Arriving with high levels of education and professional status from the sending countries, this group encountered blocked opportunities in the U.S. labor market. They found they could not practice their previous professions in the United States because their educational credentials and qualifications did not transfer. This reality aligns with the predictions of the human capital theory employed by migration scholars. According to the human capital theory, migrants generally earn less than the native-born or find themselves in less desirable positions because the human capital acquired in countries of origin is undervalued in destination countries (Hagan, Hernández-León, and Demonsant 2015; Portes and Rumbaut 2014). Historians Marilyn Halter and Violet Showers Johnson's account of the lives and experiences of West African immigrants from the late 1960s to the present day revealed that this devaluation of African-derived qualifications has long been typical, and that U.S. employers have come to treat these credentials with "contempt and mistrust" (Halter and Showers Johnson 2014, 85). Faced with a process of deskilling because of the rejection of their credentials, participants in this study embraced care work as a new livelihood strategy, taking what Halter and Showers Johnson have termed "occupational detours" in their transition to life in the United States.

Amos Ngo exemplifies the third group. Amos was as an aeronautic engineer in Cameroon but took an "occupational detour" into care work after he moved to the United States in the early nineties. He was an active critic of the Francophone government's marginalization of the English-speaking minority, of which he is a member. He arrived in Dallas, Texas, on a visitor's visa to attend an academic conference and sought political asylum in the United States because of the persecution he had faced in his home country, leaving his wife and children behind. Amos went through years of uncertainty while he waited for his asylum case to be adjudicated. This meant he could work only by petitioning for a temporary work permit that he had to renew annually. Even though he had authority to work, albeit temporarily, employers dismissed his educational credentials and previous work experience. Plagued with the problems arising from his liminal immigration status and by the lack of acceptable credentials, he began work in Dallas in the informal gardening/landscaping sector and, later, selling phone cards to his coethnics. Finding it difficult to make ends meet, he then moved to the DC-area, where he could count on the support of his Cameroonian friends. While in DC, he became a home health aide, working in the homes of mostly lower-income African American patients.

Amos struggled as a home health aide. He despaired because of the intimate aspects of the job (bathing, cleaning, and dealing with body fluids, excreta, etc.). He also felt disrespected, both by the people for whom he cared and by the U.S. society that did not recognize him as an engineer. Even though Amos suffered from the loss of status that came with moving from an engineer to an entry-level care worker, he remained in the United States because of the political situation back home. Many study participants, like Amos, remained in the United States

despite working in low-status occupations in the early years and enduring difficulties, because they could earner higher incomes than they did in their home
countries. Life in the United States also sometimes granted them political stability and safety, as well as other amenities they lacked back home, such as access to
satisfactory health care, access to a U.S. education for their children, etc. Other
scholars have found that the shame of failure and the fear of returning home with
little to show for their sojourns also force West Africans to remain in low-status
occupations (Miraftab 2016).

After a few years, and increasingly disillusioned with his job as a home health
aide, Amos quit and became a car mechanic for a large national car repair chain.
He did this job only briefly before he heard that the owner of a small home care
staffing agency, a fellow Cameroonian, was looking for a manager. He occupied
this role when I met him. He said of the agency's decision to hire him even though
he did not have any formal managerial experience or business training in the
United States: "They found out that having worked in the field, in my caliber as
someone who has read a lot, they found out that I was a good fit for the job and
that was how I was offered the job to come and run the agency." Unlike U.S.
employers who dismissed Amos's African-earned credentials, because of "ignorance or arrogance," according to historians Halter and Showers Johnson, a fellow
African recognized and rewarded his qualifications as well as the life experiences
he brought with him. Working in a supervisory role as opposed to direct care
work was congruent with Amos's perception of appropriate masculinity. Being a
manager also helped resolve some of the class conflict and contradiction that
troubled him when he had worked as a home health aide.

Amos's caring trajectory shows that entry-level jobs in the care industry
become an entry point into the formal U.S. labor market. Faced with structural
barriers and obstacles in continuing their previous career paths in professional
sectors of the economy or encountering blocked opportunities in U.S. society,
middle-class West Africans sought employment in sectors that willingly receive
newly arrived immigrants, such as entry-level health care positions. The experiences of these immigrants fall in line with the theory of segmented labor markets, which suggests that advanced economies produce an unlimited number of
jobs at the lower end of the occupational structure that are difficult to fill with
native-born workers but are attractive to newly arrived immigrant workers
(Piore 1979; Portes and Rumbaut 2014). In addition to little competition from
native-born workers, entry jobs in the health and long-term care sectors also
lacked, from the perspective of subjects, an exorbitant credentialing process. For
instance, HHAs and CNAs typically must train for six to eight weeks. Amos confirmed this experience when he stated:

All these Africans find themselves in the nursing field because it is what is easily
and readily available; it is something you can easily navigate in. If you want a job

at a general bank or whatever, they will ask you to go to university for so many years, if you want a teaching job, you will have to go to school. So, sometimes you look at the process it takes. Back home, you have to send money back home, so you do what you see. I got into home health aide business because I had no option. I needed to work and that was what I could easily grab or easily get into. You do the course, you come out, go to an agency and they give you a client and you start working.

As Amos's comments illustrate, many West Africans, especially those with family responsibilities in the United States and transnationally, felt that direct care work was one of the few options available to them. While entering in the lower-tier occupational categories, as HHAs or CNAs for instance, some of my research participants, such as Sarah discussed earlier, sought and were successful in gaining further educational credentials in the field. Additional years of schooling ranged from two to four years to become an LPN or RN. Even though these are the normative length of completion for these degrees, many of the nurses and others on the professional track in the health care field took many more years (five years on average) to complete an associate degree, as they combined working full time, family responsibilities both in the United States and back home, and financial constraints while simultaneously taking classes part-time. Completing these further credentials led to higher incomes and, as we shall see later, more opportunities for professional advancement and satisfaction.

The concentration of West African immigrants in direct care work also reflects processes of racialization that construct immigrants, women, and people of color as ideal for low-wage or undesirable care occupations, as well as racial discrimination that limits their entry into more prestigious and desirable occupations (Coe 2019; Covington-Ward 2017; Halter and Showers Johnson 2014; Showers 2015a, 2015b, 2018). Anthropologist Cati Coe also recognized home care work as "a portal" to the U.S. economy for African migrants, especially women, but also described it as leading to "a dead end" (Coe 2019, 42). She acknowledged that nursing and other health care licensures are routes to higher pay and higher status but obscured the experience of people like Sarah, who went from CNA to nurse, or cases like Amos's, where it became possible to capitalize on experience in home health care or leverage premigration experience and credentials to find a professional job in the field. The distinguishing factors among individuals like Sarah, Amos, and other subjects of this book that allowed for upward mobility were that they had premigration class privilege, (almost all the participants in this research were born into middle-class to upper middle-class families, and the ones who came from less privileged backgrounds had achieved professional success and middle-class status before they migrated). They had access to formal education (often a college degree) before migration. They migrated from urban centers (often the capital city of their countries) and, perhaps, had lesser obligations to care financially for large, extended families compared to those from more rural backgrounds.[2] Many, like Nelson and Musu mentioned previously, had not started families before they migrated or had support from family members in the home countries when they left children behind. A few, as we will see later, sent U.S.-born children to be cared for by relatives in the home country, thus saving on the exorbitant costs of childcare in the United States. In addition to transnational family resources, as chapter 1 showed, they had access to social capital via their family members already settled in the United States and the presence of West African-owned businesses that could employ some when they had encountered obstacles or provide them with a pathway to professional status.

Unlike Amos, Marcus Jean, another immigrant from Cameroon, did find work in his field after migration. However, achieving this feat was not without difficulties. A high school teacher in Cameroon, Marcus found, at first, that employers dismissed his prior experience, seeking proof of U.S.-based experience. He also faced "African-origin discrimination," contempt for and racist animus toward Africans that, in this case, manifested as prejudice against his accent. When he finally obtained a job as a teacher, he encountered obstacles, as the students complained they could not understand his accent. For his part, Marcus described the high school students he encountered as "rude, uncooperative, and lacking in good learning habits." Discouraged in the classroom and with his goals unfulfilled, Marcus decided to train as a nurse, following the advice of his Cameroonian friends and acquaintances. He kept his job as a teacher as well as a part-time job as a security guard he had taken to help pay his nursing tuition and went to nursing school at night. In entering nursing, his ambition was not to provide direct bedside care but, rather, to become a labor broker or recruiter in health care. He believed a nursing degree and knowledge of the field would help him be successful as a recruiter. He told me he had entered the home care industry because he had seen other Cameroonians who had been successful in the role, who were providing for their families in the United States and in Cameroon. This suggests the influence of West African immigrant ethnic networks in shaping choices such as Marcus's.

THE ROLE OF AFRICAN IMMIGRANT NETWORKS

When I met Marcus, he was working as a visiting nurse for two West African-owned agencies. He had worked in a hospital for two years before becoming a home nurse. His job involved visiting the homes of prospective patients and doing a needs assessment to determine whether that patient required agency services. He also visited the homes of current patients once a month to supervise the home health aide working in the home and to do a continued needs assessment. This was to ensure that the agency remained compliant with the requirements specified by the government-funded Medicaid program. In addition, he also had obtained his objective of becoming, in his words, a "nurse staffer" or "independent contractor," recruiting staff to fill vacancies in home care.

As a "nurse staffer," Marcus had a contract to provide the agencies with a ready pool of workers. He told me he ensured that the individuals he hired met the minimum requirements for employment, including citizenship and residency requirements and background checks in keeping with federal regulations and the regulations set by the hiring agency. The agency paid the aides, who might work four to eight hours a day, directly from their payroll, while he received a commission for his labor brokering services. Marcus's own social and ethnic networks were vital in this respect, as he tapped into these networks to hire workers. The aides, for their own part, often worked with more than one agency to cobble together enough paid hours to make a living, thus feeding the need for the services of people like Marcus.

As Marcus described it, in addition to recruitment, he maintained familiarity with all the patients for whom his aides provided care. He also checked in with the aides he recruited to make sure they were physically present at work and performing their duties. He monitored any problematic situations, acting as a liaison between the hiring agency and his recruits. His personal connections to them often made these interactions smoother. He reported any problems that arose, and any discrepancies between his staff's account and the patients' account of care to the hiring agency.

Given the level of oversight Marcus provided, when I asked Marcus about how many aides were working for the agencies he had recruited, I expected him to say about a dozen. I was shocked when he retorted "About ninety." I asked him whether he conducted business from an office, and he smiled wryly, saying, "My office is my car and my cell phone." He told me that "his" staff were predominantly Cameroonian and Nigerian. The nationality of his aides reflected the fact that he pulled mostly from his own ethnic network. The pool of Nigerian workers was a result of contacts he made while he worked for a previous hiring agency. Contacts from that agency continued to recommend aides who needed additional work outside of the hours offered by their agency.

Marcus's caring trajectory shows the strength of social networks that African immigrants had formed around care and the embeddedness of West African ethnic networks within webs and circuits of care. In addition to the interpersonal ties within networks of family, friends, colleagues, and acquaintances that prompted Marcus to pursue work in health care and that he drew on to recruit workers, these networks also included organizational ties established through recruitment agencies and health care provision businesses sanctioned and supported by the DC government. As Marcus's case suggests, formal (organizational) and informal (interpersonal) ties within networks often meshed and fused.

For some research participants, the influence of immigrant networks was felt even before they came to the United States. Immigrants already established in the United States, especially those who become successful as nurses, regaled family members back home with tales of their success in America in general and in health care. Even low-status health care workers could craft a narrative of success through the remittances they sent to family back home and, as geographer JoAnn McGregor found among Zimbabwean care workers in the U.K., by sending money but conveniently leaving out the details of work duties performed.

In some cases, care pioneers within West African immigrant networks placed newly arrived immigrants in health care positions shortly after they arrived. Fatima Kamara, a Sierra Leonean immigrant described:

> Each time from back home [in Sierra Leone] I always hear that if you sweep the floor, you will be paid money, you wash plates at the restaurant, I heard all those stories. . . . So, I came and the way we thought, it was not that way [referencing dashed expectations]. It was not even easy to get a job and the only way everybody said is nursing and most of my friends were certified nursing assistants. Usually, they take you to those nursing homes they train you but if you don't want to wait you can pay [for training]. Fortunately, I came with some money . . . cash and at that time, I haven't got any papers to work and through the help of one of my uncle's wife she gave me a job where she was working, and I was working there at night.

Fatima's aunt was working in the home of an American older adult in an informal care arrangement. She arranged for Fatima to work in the home, and together they provided round-the-clock care, with each of them working twelve-hour shifts. Due to Fatima's undocumented status at the time, she could not seek a more formal arrangement with regularized working hours and payroll procedures. As sociologist Evelyn Nakano Glenn describes, such "gray markets" are common in "global cities." She describes "a vibrant underground economy" that coexists with "a booming corporation-dominated formal economy" for care, noting that affluent middle-class families were increasingly seeking household help and home care for their parents through such gray markets (Glenn 2010, 177). Fatima later married a U.S. citizen and having obtained legal status, went to nursing school part-time while continuing to work as a nursing aide, but the network that provided her first job had been vital to her initial survival.

For other immigrants, their initiation into care work began upon arrival. Yenoh Sesay, a master's degree-holding nurse from Sierra Leone, was particularly conscious of the role ethnic networks played in siphoning new arrivals into the health care industry. She said: "In the Sierra Leonean community, even in the asylum cases, [if] you know of one lawyer everybody will be with that lawyer. . . . I remember there was one Nigerian lawyer, his name was Cooper. All of us went to Cooper. So likewise, when you come [to the United States] in the [19]90s [Sierra Leoneans] had no other profession but nursing."

Like Amos and Marcus, Yenoh had a professional background, having worked in a management position at a government agency in Sierra Leone. Yenoh explained that she wanted to continue in business administration or public service, but people in her family and friendship network discouraged her, telling her she could not get a job or additional schooling without a green card, and saying her accent would also be a barrier. "I mean," she said of her networks, "they will discourage you from doing any other thing." She acquiesced and become a registered nurse after receiving her green card. She later earned a master's degree. The idea that nursing jobs were readily available, and that the health care field was open to absorbing immigrants, even African immigrants, was recurrent in the interviews I conducted. This construction of nursing as desirable and open was powerfully captured in this statement made by Yenoh: "In nursing, whether you are green, whether you are Black, whether you are short, whether you are fat, whether you are young, whether you are old—there are nurses who are seventy years old still working. Other professions, no. [Meaning this is not the case in other professions]. They need your skills, they need you, and so they hire you."

Indeed, several nurses, when asked to describe the ethnic/racial makeup of their wards/units in cosmopolitan Washington, DC, described them as "like the United Nations," referring to the presence of ethnic diversity that is uncommon in many other high status professions, and in the nursing profession nationally, which is dominated by white women (American Association of Colleges of Nursing, 2019). Care pioneers within West African ethnic networks thus steered their members toward a field that was likely to absorb them, even if one had to start at the bottom to get a foothold in the industry. Younger women typically emphasized the professional rewards of nursing. For example, a young Sierra Leonean nurse said:

> The reason why we do it [nursing] is because it's . . . a sustainable career path. In the sense that you can always find a job. You will never go out of a job. You can go anywhere in the world and practice. You can do almost anything with nursing. That's one thing people don't realize; they just think it's cleaning crap. . . . You can be a research nurse, a nurse educator, administrative nurse, a charge nurse, you can do business with nursing selling equipment. You can be a psychiatric nurse, you can be a pediatric nurse, you can be a cardiac nurse, you can be a maternity nurse. You can do anything with it.

Similarly, historians Marilyn Halter and Violet Johnson have documented the role of West African ethnic networks and institutions in the United States and transnationally in advertising the possibility of upward social mobility and gaining material success through nursing. They describe a pattern in which West African communities throughout the United States, as well as in countries in West Africa, share an understanding that nurses in the United States are quite prosperous, owning expensive cars and luxurious homes. They write that it is common to show visitors to such communities the "elegant houses of nurses in affluent parts of Bowie, Maryland, [a DC suburb]." Further, they report that *African Abroad* [a print newspaper that caters to the African immigrant population] frequently offers illustrative accounts of nurses, invariably women, who throw spectacular housewarming parties to "present their mansions and give thanks for prosperity" (Halter and Showers Johnson 2014, 93–94). Thus, the picture was clearly painted that immigrants could aspire to prosperity, attain the American dream, and redeem lost status if one could join the ranks of professional health care workers. (Figure 2.1 depicting a Nigerian nurse who had attained a doctorate in nursing practice symbolizes the pinnacle of the American dream in the minds of these immigrants.)

Feminist sociologist Miliann Kang, writing about Korean immigrants and their concentration in the beauty industry (nail industry) in New York City, also suggests the importance of immigrant ethnic networks in channeling migrants into particular jobs, as ethnic networks were central in determining the labor market trajectories of Korean immigrants. Such networks not only provide crucial connections but also "normalize work that might otherwise be stigmatized" (Kang 2010, 47). Sociologist Pawan Dhingra, who focused on Indian immigrant motel owners, also notes that ethnic networks, in particular extended family, prove "an invaluable resource of information and inspiration" (Dhingra 2012, 86). Indeed, the literature on immigration in the United States has long accounted for the role of immigrant ethnic networks in facilitating the migration of ethnic groups, aiding their entry into the U.S. labor market, especially into specific industries. Scholars have termed the resulting concentration of an ethnic group in an area of the labor market as the formation of an ethnic niche of employment within the given industry. Newcomers learn about job information, settlement advice, business opportunities, etc. when embedded within these ethnic networks (Bashi 2007; Dhingra 2012; Kang 2010; Kasinitz and Vickerman 2001; Poros 2011; Vickerman 1999; Waldinger 1996; Waldinger and Lichter 2003). The activation and operation of these immigrant networks are elucidated theoretically through the migration systems theory (Massey 1999).

Based on workers' accounts, I found that West African ethnic networks in metropolitan Washington, DC, operated in three major ways. The first was that ethnic networks, family networks specifically, motivated and/or facilitated an immigrant's entry into the United States by sponsoring their migration. As described in chapter 1, several study participants arrived in the United States as family-sponsored migrants to join family members who were already present in the United States. Some others arrived using various temporary visa categories, such as student and tourist visas, and stayed with family members or friends while they settled into society.

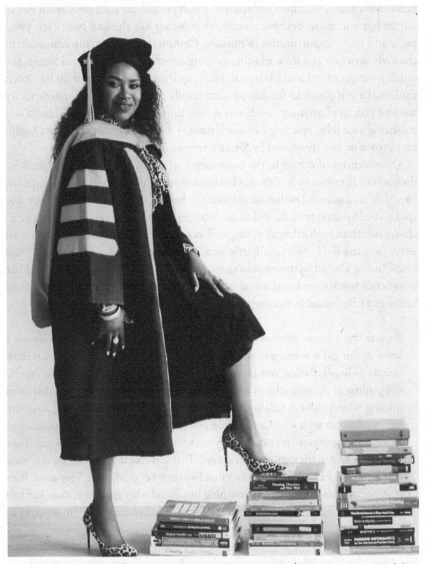

FIGURE 2.1. Graduation photo with doctor of nursing practice. (Photo courtesy Omolola Akolo, MSN, DNP. Photographer: Kesnia Pro Photography.)

Second, immigrant ethnic networks provided information about the health care field as a viable career option for newly arrived immigrants. Sometimes the influence of networks was direct, as when care pioneers told individual immigrants about the field and urged them to train as nurses or other health care workers. Claudia Johnson, a young immigrant from Sierra Leone, had migrated to the United States as a young adult to pursue a bachelor's degree in business administration. A year into her studies, she reported, an aunt convinced her to switch her studies to become a nurse, convincing her she had better job prospects and more opportunities in nursing. Completing her nursing education in the early nineties, at a time of acute nursing shortages in the United States, she quickly was recruited into a hospital. Her employer also petitioned for her green card, making it possible for her to successfully transition from her temporary student visa to permanent residence. At the time of the interview, Claudia was balancing two jobs, splitting her work time at a DC-area hospital and a health care provision facility owned by Sierra Leoneans.

Observations of others in the community who had made successful lives for themselves as nurses or health care business owners also influenced participants, like Marcus, discussed earlier, to get into the field. A few U.S.-trained nurses also spoke about seeing friends and acquaintances from their home countries (e.g., classmates from high school), doing well as nurses and that prompted their own entry into the field. Maryam Barrie was in the category of migrants who had come to the United States as teenagers. She is now a registered nurse, and her experience was somewhat unusual in that she credits a later arrival to the United States as a role model in nursing:

> So, one day a friend of mine just came from Sierra Leone, 2000/2001. Before I knew it, this girl was going to nursing school. She took classes at [the local community college]. Before you know it, she transferred to [the local state university], going to nursing school, and I am still there. By 2004, she graduated from nursing school and I'm still in college taking general classes. I was like, what the hell is going on with me? Until at one point, I was on academic probation, you know. I said to myself, it's not like I'm not smart, I'm smarter than this girl. They came here to America, met me in school. That was like the camel—er, the straw that broke the camel's back, the fact that I've seen her graduated. They came here to America, met me in school [meaning her friend who came later than her had surpassed her academic achievements]. I said okay, I'm going to go to school, I'm going to finish school.

Similarly, Winifred Williams, another Sierra Leonean nurse who migrated as a young adult, captured the pervasive influence of the socially constructed desirability of nursing among African (Sierra Leonean) immigrant communities when she said, "Nursing was the talk around town."

The third role of the networks was to help place individuals in the job market. As Marcus's business suggests, ethnic networks engaged in formal labor brokering processes. Also, kinship, friendship, and informal networks helped land migrants into health care jobs. Fatima, for instance, gained a job through a kin tie, while Amos found work though his Cameroonian networks. A few nurse participants also relied on informal ethnic network connections and ethnic-owned businesses for employment.

Female-centered networks were particularly instrumental in siphoning West African immigrants into health care occupations in the United States. The younger women who became health care workers, specifically nurses, in the United States reported that their mothers or other female family members had encouraged them to train as nursing assistants or home health aides as a pathway into nursing, much as Clarice, the nurse profiled in the opening of this chapter, was trying to do for her young daughter. Thelma Sankoh, a registered nurse originally from Sierra Leone, was nine when she migrated to the United States, joining her mother, who had migrated a few years before. Thelma's mother was working as a CNA and attending nursing school when Thelma arrived. At the time of our interview, Thelma's mom owned a home care and nurse staffing agency, which Thelma estimated employed over 500 aides. Thelma worked for the agency as a registered nurse, responsible for their pediatric patients. She had attended nursing school while working as an aide, and attended a local community college, where it took her five years to complete her associate degree, as she was studying part-time, on and off. When I asked her how she learned about the health care field, Thelma stated:

From my mom, because she said, "it's easier for you to get a job," so she said, "because there's always a job opportunity in nursing." She said even though I wanted to do child daycare, I can do the nursing and I can practice there [at her mom's agency], which kind of made sense. So, I felt like I was already a caring, nurturing person and so I said okay, and that's how I ended up doing nursing. At first, I started with like the home health aide certificate, I got the CNA and I worked as a home health aide.

Thelma acknowledged she was initially reluctant to become a home health aide and, later, a nurse. "I really didn't want to do it," she said. However, she reconciled her mind to the idea, because what her mother said made sense and she felt it fit her personality to do care work. The mother's actions here show how West African mother-daughter dyads operated and the influence of West African immigrant mothers in their daughters' decisions around care work. It was clear that Clarice was hoping she could have the same impact on her teenage daughter. In both cases, we see the effort of the immigrant mother in cajoling, compelling, or coercing their young daughters to enter direct care work as a pathway into nursing.

My interactions with Clarice and her daughter, Musu, mentioned earlier, who was able to get a job at a business owned by her mother's friend, and Thelma's account of her mother's actions here show how immigrant mothers shaped the caring trajectories of their immigrant 1.5 and second-generation children. Jennifer Gowon was a nurse practitioner from Nigeria in her thirties, and her mom also was a nurse. She explained that her brother became a nurse after being influenced by seeing the success of the women in his family. "My brother, like I said, I think he just saw my mom and he thought he was going to make a lot of money. So, I graduated before him and I had showed him my paycheck the first couple of months, and he was like, what? That's it, I'm going to be a nurse."

Other nurses also credited aunts and female cousins and friends whom they said convinced them to enter the health care field. These family and friendship networks also provided them with practical tips about nursing school applications, credentialing, licensing exams, etc. Paula Boateng, a licensed practical nurse from Ghana, had worked as a secretary in her home country before joining her husband, who had been an air traffic controller. While her husband found work as a cab driver, Paula initially worked in the kitchen of a nursing home and later stocked shelves at a shopping warehouse. She explained that a female relative introduced the idea of nursing as a career option: "So, my sister-in-law said, 'Auntie [a term of respect used to address an older woman regardless of actual relationship ties], since we all come from Africa, when we get here, we don't get what we want. This [nursing] is what we doing. So, if you wouldn't mind to join us.' I said 'nursing? I don't have . . . my temper is not good for nursing, so I can't do it.' So, she talked talked, talked, talked [until I was convinced]."

After she had made the decision to pursue nursing, Paula's networks were influential in providing her with career advice. When she encountered personal difficulties when she was going through a difficult pregnancy and problems with her marriage while trying to take the licensing exams, her friends advised her to downgrade from the RN certification and become an LPN first: "I talked to friends that have already finished the school, and we are talking, and they said well, if things are tough, why don't you do the LPN courses? If you think that the RN course is too much, you can do the LPN courses. So, friends where I used to work, and we talked, and that's why I changed my mind to do the LPN course." This advice was invaluable, and Paula was able to balance her role as an LPN and being a new mom.

A few nurses who trained in their home countries could draw from social networks of people they knew in nursing school who had migrated to the United States. Harriet Williams was trained as a nurse in Sierra Leone. She migrated to the United States on a visitor visa with the hope of entering nursing in the United States. When I asked her if she had information at the time about how to do that, she said:

> I did have because that my friend [a friend with whom she stayed when she just arrived] who came here before me was also a nurse. . . . and she had already come here, she had passed the exam and had become a nurse. So, I had a little bit of information as to what to do. But when I lived with her of course, you know when you come to stay with someone [alluding to fraught relationships between estab-

lished hosts and newly arrived immigrants] . . . she did help me though, in terms of finding me a job as a CNA. I started working as a CNA and I said, oh my gosh, I can't do this. I did not come here to do this.

As seen from her statement, Harriet received information about the licensing examinations that would allow for her to enter the labor force as a nurse from a Sierra Leonean friend who was also a nurse. This friend also helped her find a job in the paraprofessional sector of nursing while she was preparing to take the licensing exams. Eventually, Harriet passed her board exams and later became a nurse in a prestigious DC-area hospital.

Kate Yeboah, a nurse from Ghana, migrated to the United States as a DV Lottery winner. Friends who had migrated before her told her about nursing in the United States, and she began the time-consuming process of transferring her credentials immediately. She had been warned about the long wait for the Commission on Graduates of Foreign Nursing Schools (CGFNS, the body entrusted with validating foreign-earned credentials) to examine her transcript before she could take the licensure exam to practice in the United States, so she started the process as soon as she arrived. Another nurse said that relatives who were already in the United States told her about this requirement and she got her transcripts before she left Nigeria.

Historians Marilyn Halter and Violet Showers Johnson similarly unearthed the workings of West African female-centered networks with a focus on how they functioned in supporting nursing education. In interviews and observations conducted by Showers Johnson among West African nurses in Atlanta, she found the operation of what I term sister networks comprising Ghanaian, Nigerian, and Sierra Leonean women in Atlanta who studied for their nursing degrees in Alabama. As students, they pooled resources by carpooling to classes and sharing hotel rooms during examinations. They exchanged notes and practiced for exams together, thus making successful attainment of degrees possible.

AFRICAN IMMIGRANT ETHNIC NETWORKS AS LABOR BROKERS IN HEALTH CARE

Existing scholarship on the international migration of nurses has detailed the importance of professional networks in facilitating their entry into the nursing labor force in the United States (George 2005; Guevarra 2010; Kingma 2006; Rodriguez, 2010). For example, sociologist Sheba George (2005) found that nurses who migrated from Kerala, India, to the United States relied heavily on nursing school networks, to the extent that some of her respondents stayed with nursing school friends when they arrived in the United States instead of with relatives who had migrated before them. Anna Guevarra's research on Filipino nurse migration shows that recruitment agencies connected networks of potential migrants in the

Philippines with already-established migrants who were working in the destination countries. These networks were very useful in providing information about immigrant destinations and constructed the United States as the ideal destination for nurses. Potential migrants received significant information from such transnational networks, including advice on navigating the bureaucratic processes that aided their migrations. Other researchers have shown that state and non-state actors, such as state-run and private nursing schools in the Philippines, hospitals, and health care institutions in receiving countries, including the United States, and transnational recruitment agencies and government agencies have helped facilitate the migration of nurses and their incorporation in receiving countries' nursing labor forces (Aiken 2007; Masselink and Lee 2010; Ortiga 2014, 2017, 2018). This scholarship shows that nursing increasingly attracts people with transnational ambitions and that many people enter the profession because they wish to migrate (Banerjee 2022). The narratives outlined in this chapter suggest that interpersonal ties within immigrant ethnic networks in destination countries play as significant a role as organizational ties within professional networks. Participants relied on such networks for assistance with sponsoring their migrations; housing in their initial years; knowledge of the health care field that sparked their desires; information about licensing and credentialing procedures; and assistance with job market placement.

Much has been made of the cyclical but long-standing shortage of care workers in the United States, and the drums of panic have sounded as to who will provide care for the increasing numbers of vulnerable older adults. The story that has not being given as much attention is the story of women and men who leave their home countries for various reasons and arrive in the United States through established migration channels made possible by U.S. immigration policies. They arrive just in time to provide one of the most essential of duties—to take care of the sick, disabled, and frail older adults, often the poor, sick, disabled, and vulnerable. African immigrants stand out as some of the faces at the front line of care, and they also form part of the systems of brokerage located in the United States behind the provision of care. In the next chapter, I turn to the workings of formal business and entrepreneurial initiatives created by West Africans who capitalize on the social and cultural capital embedded in their ethnic networks as well as the supply of labor present in their communities to produce, repackage, and deploy African immigrants as health care workers.

3 · THE BUSINESS OF CARE
Ethnic Entrepreneurship in Care

Mrs. Hillary Johnson[1] migrated to the United States in 1967. Her husband, who was completing his undergraduate degree in Sierra Leone, joined her shortly thereafter. They both enrolled in colleges in the Washington, DC, metropolitan area and later became educators. She became a special education teacher and later worked with adults with intellectual and developmental disabilities, while he returned to school to earn a doctorate in economic development. Their first daughter was born in 1971, and as a young couple who were both students at the time, they found it difficult to arrange and pay for adequate childcare. They sent their daughter to Sierra Leone to be cared for by Mrs. Johnson's parents when she was six weeks old, where she stayed until she was four. Being separated from children to save on U.S. childcare was a sacrifice other West African immigrants I interviewed made, although, as others have found, it was more common to leave a child behind than to send a U.S.-born child back (Francisco-Menchavez 2018; Parreñas 2001, 2005, 2015). The cost-saving strategy that urban studies scholar Faranak Miraftab identified among diversity visa lottery winners from Togo, West Africa, many of whom left children in their home country, played a similar role in all these decisions (Miraftab 2016, 138).

When the Johnsons' eldest daughter returned, her parents were much more established in the United States and in a position to raise her and the two later additions to their family. The Johnsons had drawn on transnational family resources and it had worked. The arrangement also allowed Mrs. Johnson to build a career she loved. She ultimately became the program director of a vocational day program helping intellectually disabled care recipients achieve educational and developmental goals and objectives. She loved the people she cared for, with a love that she passed on to her children. As Miriam, her younger daughter recalled: "Every summer when we were out of school, we used to go and work [at the program directed by their mom]. We were very much exposed to [people with intellectual disabilities] at a very young age. I think I was about sixteen when I started working with this population."

In 1990, a representative of the Washington, DC, Department of Disability Services (DDS) approached Mrs. Johnson (as she was regularly referred to) with a proposition. They were looking for individuals and small businesses to provide care for adults with intellectual, developmental, and physical disabilities in small residential settings. Mrs. Johnson was given a contract and officially became a "provider" for the DC government. Later that year, she registered a business she called Worldwide Services Inc.[2] and served as its president. It operated as a health care company, fully licensed and accredited by the Washington, DC, Department of Disability Services and Department of Health. Using savings she and her husband had accumulated as start-up funds, she rented a house in Washington, DC, where her company provided custodial, medical, and day care support to an initial cohort of six persons.

From those modest beginnings, the company grew steadily through the years. When I met the Johnsons, Mrs. Johnson was in a state of semi-retirement. She had given up the day-to-day running of the company but came into the office about once a week. Her husband, Dr. Johnson (he had earned a PhD in the years since arriving in the United States), now retired from his job as an economist in local government, also dropped in periodically. All three of their adult children had leadership roles in the company. Malaika, who held a law degree, was the vice president of the company and oversaw its operations. She ensured that they complied with local and federal regulations, which included interacting with at least five DC government agencies and departments as well as independent agencies that dealt with the welfare and legal issues pertaining to individuals with intellectual disabilities, many of whom were wards of the state. Miriam, a registered nurse, was the director of nursing (DON). She supervised the registered and licensed practical nurses employed by the company and coordinated the medical care for their care recipients. Kareem, their brother, was the training coordinator for the company. He led a small team responsible for coordinating the orientation and training of new staff members and providing in-service or "refresher" training for current workers according to the bureaucratic, ethical, and professional standards set by DDS. For example, to become certified as direct support professionals, trainees had to complete a requisite number of hours of online instruction and receive certifications on topics such as "use of adaptive equipment," "abuse, neglect, and exploitation," and "safety and universal precautions." While new recruits bore the cost of the online training and organized their certifications on their own, Kareem and his team were responsible for orienting new employees to the agency and coordinating ongoing trainings on issues covered in the DSP training, as well as other policy issues

All the Johnson siblings described the business as a "family business," and routinely described their staff as part of the "Worldwide family." Not all the ties in the company "family" were fictive, either. Spending significant time in the agency, I learned, for example, that a registered nurse working for the company had a stepmother who was also a staff member. An administrator's ex-partner, with whom she shared a son, happened to be the brother of one of the senior staff members. There also was a husband-and-wife team on staff. Through blood, official, and fictive kinship ties, they really were the "Worldwide family." Mrs. Johnson had become the ultimate care pioneer, or central actor, in an organizational network that linked members of her family and many other West Africans (Sierra Leoneans) through their labor in disability support.

Worldwide provided nursing/clinical, physical, vocational, and recreational services for adults (many of them older adults) with severe physical, developmental, and intellectual disabilities.[3] Some of their care recipients also had diagnoses of mental illness and other chronic health conditions. Worldwide provided occupational and speech therapy, nutrition, and social work services as needed. A physician, also a Sierra Leonean immigrant, worked with them on a contract basis as a medical consultant. They employed five full-time RNs and twenty-two LPNs. They also employed over 200 direct care and supervisory staff. The majority were DSPs. House managers supervised the DSPs and oversaw the residential care homes they operated; QIDPs supervised the house managers and coordinated legal affairs, medical appointments, etc. for their care recipients; and case managers supervised the intake of new clients at a day program they organized. Case managers and QIDPs also coordinated care with other providers, such as DDS service coordinators and social workers.

Worldwide cared for a total population of 189 persons. Among these, eighty-three lived in the organization's twenty-four residential care facilities, which ranged in size from two-person apartments to larger homes that housed up to six people, and included a set of "medically fragile" homes for those needing the most intensive care. The services they provided included twenty-four-hour custodial care; medical services such as medication management and coordinating medical visits; three meals a day; and skilled nursing care for care receivers with chronic conditions. The company website described the residential support as "designed to assist each person in acquiring, retaining, and improving self-care, daily living, adaptive and other skills needed to reside successfully as part of their community." They also ran a day program serving 106 persons. My observations suggest that claims made in their company website were accurate: "Day services are provided in the most integrated, inclusive setting allowing for as much meaningful interaction with non-disabled persons as practicable. Services are delivered consistent with the interest, strengths, needs and preferences of the person being supported."

Worldwide's main office was situated along a major avenue in the nation's capital. It shared the top floor of a large, two-story office/retail plaza with one other organization, a legal aid service for low-income DC residents. The bottom floor and immediate surroundings of the building housed a large shopping plaza with small retail businesses, all mainstays of low-income urban scape, including fast-food establishments Subway and Popeyes; the furniture leasing company, Rent-A-Center; a beauty supply store; and Save a Lot, a discount grocery store chain.

In this chapter, I explore how West African immigrants have formed businesses like Worldwide that capitalize on the labor of their coethnics and a racialized market in health and long-term care to cater to some of the most underserved populations. The pages that follow will review the structural landscape that created the opening that West Africans like the Johnsons have seized upon to become care providers in disability and home care. I then provide an ethnographic lens into the world of Worldwide and two other businesses, showing West African immigrants as providers of care who strive to provide services that meet the criteria and regulations set by state, federal, and district regulatory and oversight bodies. I reveal how these West African health care entrepreneurs expressed their motivations to enter the business of care and how they viewed their obligations to the people they cared for and their staff. Noting their triumphs and travails in navigating the DC bureaucratic care landscape, I show that some of these businesses, as exemplified by Worldwide, strive to provide compassionate and professional care despite many constraints. The chapter ends by shedding light on these entrepreneurs as employers responsible for repackaging, transforming, and deploying coethnics as care workers, and thus sustaining the West African labor market niche in care.

THE PRIVATIZATION AND DEINSTITUTIONALIZATION OF CARE

The Johnsons' caring trajectory intersects with two broader historical and structural changes that took hold in the U.S. health care landscape starting in the 1950s and solidifying in the 1980s: the privatization and deinstitutionalization of care. The federal government and individual states have, increasingly, leased the responsibility for health and long-term care delivery to market forces and outside entities, while still providing some of the funding streams available for the poor, those with limited assets, and individuals age sixty-five and above (Boris and Klein 2012; Cranford 2020; Glenn 2010; Osterman 2017). The privatization of long-term care aligns with neoliberal ideologies that dictate that "governments should steer and not row the ship of state" and that "rather than provide services, government should ensure that services are provided and do so through supporting competition and markets" (Armstrong and Armstrong 2019, 17).

Medicaid and Medicare, two of the major sources of federal and state welfare funding for health and long-term care, were established in the 1960s to finance health care for the poor (Medicaid) and adults sixty-five years of age and over (Medicare). Medicare prescribes care based on a medical model and covers only in-patient hospital care and/or thirty days of skilled nursing care in a facility such as a nursing home (Boris and Klein 2012; Buch 2018). Medicare also reimburses for the cost of short-term (up to a hundred days) rehabilitative care in the home after a hospital stay of at least three nights (Coe 2019; Rodriquez 2014). Medicare has a higher a reimbursement rate than Medicaid (Osterman 2017; Rodriquez 2014), and reimbursement rates from private insurance companies are even higher.

Whereas Medicare is entirely federally funded, Medicaid is jointly funded by the federal government and individual states. The latter allows for a broader range of care, including long-term habilitative services[4] and skilled nursing and personal care services in the home. Medicaid also offers a waiver program that allows states to provide benefits not normally covered by Medicaid if such provision will prevent the individual from being institutionalized (Buch 2018). Accordingly, all states and the District of Columbia offer home-based health care services, with most operating under these various waivers. In this way, Medicaid pushes the responsibility of long-term care away from public and state institutions onto private agencies who broker care in the home, and to unpaid family caregivers who address gaps in care (Buch 2018; Cranford 2020; Glenn 2010). To be eligible for Medicaid, recipients must meet certain medical and financial requirements. These include having few assets and limited income,[5] making most middle-class adults ineligible except in cases where individuals "spend down their assets" to qualify (Rodriquez 2014; Schweid 2021; Osterman 2017; Stacey 2011).

In addition to federal and state medical funding policies, other actors, such as the independent living movement of non-elderly adults with physical disabilities, have played a role in the deinstitutionalization of care and the shift toward home-based or community-based care (Boris and Klein 2012; Buch 2018; Cranford 2020; Glenn 2010; Osterman 2017). Since the 1960s, politically organized disability activists have lobbied to get laws passed requiring states to provide services and accommodations that will allow disabled children and adults to live independently in their communities. They stressed the positive and empowering aspects of deinstitutionalization of the elderly, the ill, and the disabled (Boris and Klein 2012; Buch 2018; Osterman 2017). Disability advocates in California, for instance, argued for the closure of institutions and an elimination of the "agency model" that allows for state governments to contract service organizations who then hire workers. They fought for the independent provider model, in which the care recipient has the authority to hire, fire, and supervise their own care workers (Cranford 2020).

The neoliberal privatization of welfare and the growing rejection of institutional long-term care facilities, such as state mental health facilities, institutions for the physically and intellectually disabled, and, more recently, nursing homes, have opened the door for various for-profit and nonprofit entities to enter the market for home care, or hybridized alternatives such as small residential care homes or group homes. State agencies administering federal and state-subsidized programs have contracted health and personal care services for vulnerable older adults and the disabled to outside entities, including for-profit businesses. Some of these businesses are small, family-owned operations like Worldwide, but "large corporate agencies, chains, and franchises with a national or regional presence" are not unusual (Coe 2019, 17). These providers depend on both federal and state government funds and private insurance dollars (Buch 2018; Coe 2019; Cranford 2020; Glenn 2010; Nazareno 2018; Osterman 2017; Rodriquez, 2014; Stacey 2011). Reflecting the growth of the private sector in care, a study by the Centers for Disease Control and Prevention reported that there were 12,200 home health agencies and 28,900 residential care communities operating nationwide in 2016, 80 percent of which were operated by for-profit entities (Harris-Kojetin et al. 2019).

The for-profit sector of home and institutional care has become stratified and increasingly bifurcated into a "two-tier system" that serves different socioeconomic segments of the market. At the higher end are agencies that offer premium services for affluent individuals who pay for care privately through savings, long-term care insurance, or other arrangements. At the opposite end are home care agencies that serve individuals who rely mostly on allowances from Medicaid or other government-subsidized programs (Coe 2019; Glenn 2010; Nazareno 2018). Worldwide is part of this latter segment. The Johnsons also are part of a growing pool of racial minority immigrant entrepreneurs who care for underserved populations. In one of the first studies of this group of immigrant entrepreneurs, sociologist Jennifer Nazareno (2018) has drawn attention to the experiences of Filipina entrepreneurs in Southern California who opened small-scale residential care facilities, filling a gap in the labor market for providers for the poor who suffer from severe mental health conditions. She describes such immigrant businesses as "welfare state replacements" that take over the care of the poor and those segments of care recipients displaced by the closure of public state mental health hospitals resulting from austere welfare policies.

Likewise, West African immigrants in metropolitan Washington, DC, have entered the long-term care and health care provision market as entrepreneurs by catering to impoverished individuals with severe intellectual and physical disabilities and those diagnosed with chronic mental and physical health conditions. Indeed, the Johnsons' clientele were almost exclusively Medicaid beneficiaries, and most were African Americans. The major source of their funding was a home- and community-based Medicaid waiver program designed to enable individuals with disabilities to remain in their homes and communities. After over twenty years in the industry, however, the Johnsons had become a key local player in disability support. As second-generation immigrants, Mrs. Johnson's children had the requisite cultural capital to deal effectively with African American care recipients and their families as well as policymakers and administrators in the government disability support and nonprofit bureaucracy in that area, who were mostly white women and African American men and women. Malaika, the company's

VP, held leadership roles in various DDS committees and task forces. In this way, she had the eyes and ears of the powers that be in the Washington, DC, disability support and long-term care landscape. This made Worldwide a leader among other providers of disability support.

ETHNIC ENTREPRENEURSHIP IN CARE

The Johnsons stood apart from the other West African-owned health care businesses I observed, due to their longevity and the leadership of the immigrant second generation. Many other businesses were owned and operated by first-generation immigrants and operated smaller-scale operations, as judged by their office space and number of staff.[6] However, most of these other businesses relied on the same Medicaid waiver program as Worldwide. Some also operated both day programs and residential care facilities for adults with physical and intellectual disabilities, but many operated as small-scale home care agencies[7] catering to vulnerable older adults or people with chronic health conditions and/or physical disabilities and thus did not have the range of professional care workers employed at Worldwide. These agencies hired mostly paraprofessional home care staff who assisted older adults with activities of daily living (ADLs, such as eating, bathing, toileting) and instrumental activities of daily living (IADLs, such as cooking and cleaning). They also hired home care nurses (RNs or LPNs) who established a plan of care under the direction of a physician and sometimes in conjunction with other professionals, such as a nutritionist. The nurses supervised the direct care workers and provided basic nursing care (e.g., wound care, diabetes management, managing catheters, etc.) for home-based patients. The agencies relied on doctor and social worker referrals, Medicaid, DDS, and private insurance company referrals, word of mouth, and individual's requests for their services. An administrator I interviewed told me that current home health aides were one of their most effective recruiters of clients. For instance, since many aides worked in apartment buildings and multiple-family homes in urban neighborhoods, they sometimes referred potential clients they met in the laundry rooms and other shared spaces of buildings. Also, care recipients of in-home services told their family members and neighbors with similar needs about the agency's services. Those referred then came into the office seeking the paperwork to request services.

While many of these agencies were West African-owned, a few I came across were owned by East Africans (Tanzanians and Kenyans mostly). For the most part, businesses were dominated by a single national group, but I did find some variation, including a few East Africans working for West Africans. As shown in chapter 2, informal immigrant social and ethnic networks helped siphon coethnics into these businesses. There were also a small minority of African American direct care workers and nonclinical staff, such as human resources managers.

Like Worldwide, many agencies occupied offices in low-income urban neighborhoods, although a few could be found in recently gentrified or gentrifying neighborhoods in Washington, DC. These tended to be housed in detached office buildings or townhouses within the city. Like Worldwide, the larger and more established agencies ran professional-looking bureaucratic organizations with reception desks that were staffed full-time, with sitting areas and bustling offices, where it was usual to see administrators in business casual attire and direct care staff in health care worker uniforms or "scrubs" engaged in a flurry of activity. They had designated conference rooms or spaces where new recruits were oriented to their agency and where current workers received instructional modules on various aspects of care mandated by DDS and DOH. Many other agencies operated smaller office spaces, two or three rented rooms within large office complexes concentrated in the outskirts of Washington, DC., and across the border into Maryland. In one case, two African-owned and managed agencies were in the same office building complex, and my observations of people entering and leaving the building suggested that the other businesses in the complex largely employed and conducted business with African immigrants.

Ayo and Laura Adebayo, Nigerian immigrants who met in the United States, operated one of the agencies in that building. Ayo had taught mathematics and statistics to high school students prior to migration. He came to the United States in 1996 to study accounting in one of the DC-area universities, but a promised scholarship did not materialize, causing him to change his plans. He taught in the DC public schools for twelve years, which he said was a "horrible experience." He was reticent to discuss much more about his years as a public school teacher or his interactions with students, except to say that students who could not understand his accented English "made several attempts to frustrate me." Laura had trained as a nurse after migrating to the United States.

Like Mrs. Johnson, the Adebayos did not initially have plans to open a health care business or, in fact, any prior experience or interest in entrepreneurship. Ayo recalled that he and Laura (both fervent practicing Christians) had been inspired after attending a workshop on entrepreneurship at what he called a Christian retreat but which further discussion suggested focused as much on life skills development and networking as religion. They began to consider opening a health care business to capitalize on Laura's clinical knowledge and experience.

Just like Mrs. Hillary Johnson, the Adebayos were not much like the racial minority immigrant entrepreneurs portrayed in previous immigration scholarship. They were unlike immigrant entrepreneurs with a history of premigration orientation toward entrepreneurship (Dhingra 2012; Poros 2011) or those who went into business seeking autonomy and control of their own destinies (Dhingra 2012; Verdaguer 2009; Valdez 2008, 2011) or due to experiences of racism and discrimination in high-powered white-collar professions that led them to turn to providing professional services to coethnics (Vallejo and Canizales 2016). Indeed, these African-owned businesses largely served African Americans, not African immigrants.

At the same time, it was important to business owners like the Adebayos that they were able to employ coethnics. When I asked Ayo what motivated him and his wife to become health care entrepreneurs, he stated:

> The motivation was to get extra income, and then to help as many people as possible. Because we noticed that so many of our countrymen . . . from what we saw, notwithstanding a college degree and all that, they will still discriminate [meaning, be discriminated against]. They [meaning employers] don't want to give you the place where you belong. For whatsoever reason, the greatest [barrier] is the accent, I know. . . . Look at my case. I told you I had an account[ing] background, but to even become a cashier here, I could not. Based on that, if a person like me that came up with some level of knowledge and then it was so hard for me, then what [would] happen to the rest? And when I started my business and after seeing the plight of our fellow Nigerians, we decided that we will do all we can to help. At least if I know the person is qualified, I put the person in [give the person a job] without any prejudice.

Ayo and Laura saw an opportunity to provide employment for coethnics who might otherwise face discrimination in the labor market. Ayo framed his motivations as "helping" his coethnics. In an impassioned tone, he described highly educated Nigerian friends who had trouble finding jobs in their fields after migration. Some of his physician friends, Ayo recalled, even had to do service work in fast-food companies. Thus, Ayo and Laura saw their business as helping ameliorate some of the injustices they believed their fellow immigrants had faced in the U.S. labor market.

Rebekah Sankoh, a middle-aged Sierra Leonean registered nurse, also felt a responsibility to coethnics. Much like Laura Adebayo, she believed she could build on her experience in bedside nursing and find more opportunity in business. When I met her fourteen years after she had started her business, it was thriving. Her daughter Thelma, who Rebekah raised on her own, also worked as a registered nurse for the agency. She told me the company employed ten RNs, including herself, about fifty LPNs, and at least 500 part-time home health aides. Rebekah had surmounted considerable odds to build the business. She had a negative credit rating when she started and thus could not qualify for a business loan to cover her start-up costs. She raised the capital for her business by simultaneously working as a nurse while recruiting a few home health aides and paying their salary out of her earnings as a nurse. She ran the business out of her home. She recalled that she and Thelma sometimes went without enough to eat and bought their clothes at second-hand stores in the lean years while she was trying to grow her business. Rebekah's experiences are consistent with other minority entrepreneurs who struggle with capital both at the start-up stage and when they plan to expand their businesses (Valejo and Canizales 2016; Valdez 2011). Like Ayo, Rebecca also stated that she had started the agency to "help people that other people wouldn't employ." Also a devout Christian like the Adebayos, she used religious tones and discourses, presenting herself as being aided by God to help her fellow Sierra Leoneans, both in the United States and in the Sierra Leonean homeland. She ran a nonprofit organization that bore the same name as her agency that organized development projects in her hometown. She also was actively engaged in Sierra Leonean diasporic politics in Washington, DC.

The Johnsons also invoked similar tropes of "helping" their coethnics by providing employment, especially for newly arrived immigrants who faced obstacles in the labor market. Miriam stated of her mother's mission and goals in operating Worldwide: "Mrs. Johnson [when speaking to outsiders, the Johnson siblings referenced their mother formally] has made it very clear, because during their transition here, they get immigrants coming to America, it's not easy. So, she makes an effort to assist her community in that. You know, getting a job and giving advice and sharing that they are going through the correct process. A lot of it starts from [Worldwide]. We have people who have been working with us from the day we opened, still here."

Presenting themselves as "service oriented and charitable," West African owners of health care businesses were like the Latinx entrepreneurs in Los Angeles sociologists Jody Vallejo and Stephanie Canizales (2016) studied, although those businesses—professional services in finance, real estate, insurance, law, and public relations—catered largely to lower-income Latinx communities. By framing their business as helping "out the community" or serving "underserved Latinos" or "helping the poor," some of these entrepreneurs were simultaneously downplaying or couching their exploitation of their insider status in the Latinx market to build lucrative businesses. Similarly, West Africans like the Adebayos, Rebekah Sankoh, and the Johnsons highlighted the charitable aspects of their business endeavors, even though they had successfully capitalized on the labor available within their ethnic communities, which they extracted and, in turn, commercialized for profit. It also was noteworthy that, while they framed their work as "helping" their coethnics who would otherwise lack options in the labor market, none of the administrators or owners of health care businesses I interviewed articulated that they went into business with the motive to serve an underserved segment of the population who would otherwise struggle to find quality long-term care. In practice, however, that was precisely what they were doing.

GETTING ESTABLISHED IN CARE

Unlike Mrs. Johnson, whose pathway into entrepreneurship was relatively smooth, Ayo and Laura Adebayo, like Rebekah Sankoh, found it quite difficult to get started in business. Their first attempt, an assisted living facility[8] for older adults in Maryland, had failed. Ayo explained that they struggled to navigate the bureaucratic red tape necessary for them to be registered and fully operational. For instance, regulations dictated that they complete a Certificate of Need,[9] which they found to be a challenge. As relatively recently arrived immigrants, they found communicating with bureaucrats and fulfilling state licensing requirements difficult and frustrating. When they eventually set up the business, they failed to get an adequate number of clients that could be funded by Medicaid and other government or social security subsidized programs. Ayo said they went to doctor's offices, community events, etc., to pass out flyers to recruit service recipients. They even took out advertisements in the local papers, but they failed to enlist a substantial state-funded clientele. They also struggled to get clients who were privately funded, as he described: "Then you get most of the clients, they [pay] out of pocket. And because they pay out of pocket, they find it difficult. If they come looking at the facility, they say they will call you, [but] they will not call you. I went to all the hospitals. I have papers, flyers, I did every effort I could . . . I advertised it even in the daily newspaper but thinking that it will work."

Ayo's experiences suggest that even though there was a structural demand for care providers, first-generation African immigrants, lacking in cultural capital, struggled to navigate institutional barriers to set up businesses embedded in the mainstream economy and regulated by state institutions. While these barriers were not insurmountable, especially in the market for underserved Medicaid recipients, appealing to a privately insured and more affluent population proved more difficult.

Ayo suggested that racial discrimination played a role in their inability to attract an upmarket clientele. A study that investigated the factors that were important in choice of nursing homes among a sample of white, Black, and Latinx older adults in Boston found that factors like proximity of the facility to family members, cleanliness, appearance, feeding policies, payment policies and types of insurance accepted, and concerns about how staff treated residents were common across all racial groups. Resident/staff race concordance and culturally competent care were more important for Black and Latinx care recipients than whites. Latinx adults in that study also were interested in resident/staff language concordance. The authors conclude that "this reflects the desire to ensure social comfort and good communication for themselves or a loved one" (Hefele et al. 2016). Indeed, other studies have shown the importance of race concordance and culturally competent practice for racial minority patients. Some studies have argued that previous experiences with racism in patient/provider interactions shape these preferences (Aronson, et al. 2013; LaVeist, Nuru-Jeter, and Jones 2003; Sacks 2019). However, as a dominant group, whites also may expect owners of small residential care facilities to have good communication and the cultural facility to interact adequately with care recipients and their family members, and they may not have this confidence with immigrants, especially non-white ones. The difficulties the Adebayos faced elucidate how the race, class, ethnicity/national origin status of owners/administrators and facility, and funding type intersect in shaping preferences for care.

Ayo and Laura started their current business in home health care after attending another conference; this time, a conference for owners of assisted living facilities. A friend, also an African immigrant, who also was attending the conference, advised them to try a home health care business. Unlike their first venture, in which they tried to provide care for adults in Maryland, they decided to limit their services to pediatric clients and young adults up to twenty-one years of age with special needs, and to provide care for Washington, DC, residents. While Ayo credited his friend for helping them come to this decision, limiting their services to children and young adults made sense since Laura had worked as a pediatric nurse for many years. In 2005, they registered a home health care agency, Larayo Health Services, Inc. They provided skilled services such as physical therapy, occupational therapy, speech therapy, and social work, in addition to nursing and personal care services. Most of their clients were beneficiaries of a specialized Medicaid program for children with special needs who received Supplementary Social Security Income. The program coordinates physical, mental, developmental, and behavioral health care services for children and young adults up to twenty-five years, utilizing their networks of over 2,000 providers. Rebekah Sankoh reported that her pediatric clients were almost exclusively enrolled in that program, as well.

Laura and Ayo had been in business for about seven years when I spoke to Ayo, but they still had difficulties in managing their home care business. Ayo said, "Even up to now it's horrible." In other words, after surmounting the obstacles in establishing their business, they still had trouble navigating complicated government requirements. Ayo found his interactions with bureaucrats particularly stressful. To maintain their business and to continue to qualify for state subsidies, Ayo and Laura maintained aggressive advertising efforts to get care recipients. They worked with private insurance companies and doctors' offices that provided them with client information drawn from their databases. The Johnsons did not have similar problems in getting established and in recruiting recipients of care. As Miriam, the DON, told me:

> We don't look for it. Business comes to us. We've been here long enough. We provide excellent care. It's a family-run business, so we're on the ground, and our interest, obviously is there. When you're dealing with human lives, your approach has got to be a little different. It's not a business you do and just kind of stay remotely and let people run it. No, you really have to have that thumbprint on it. It's a family. I have cousins who work here. I have friends who work here. We definitely are the [Worldwide] family as we like to put it.

Worldwide's established reputation in the industry meant that they did not have shortages of staff or care recipients. Miriam also claimed that their interest and investment in caring for others set them apart. However, it was easy to observe that the collegiality the Johnsons had established with DC government officials and disability support bureaucrats, as well as their longer experience in the industry compared to the Adebayos, had an impact.

"IF YOU DON'T DOCUMENT IT, IT DIDN'T HAPPEN": NAVIGATING THE REGULATORY REGIME IN DISABILITY SUPPORT

Nonetheless, the Johnsons, like the other West African immigrant owner/ administrators, found keeping up with the state, federal, and district regulations and requirements to maintain their provider licenses difficult. The requirement that they document every aspect of care provided to be eligible for government-funded reimbursements and prove they were not committing Medicaid fraud created significant stress. When I asked Miriam what the most challenging aspect of her job was, she said, "Crossing your I's, crossing your T's and ensuring that the documentation is consistent to what we're doing on a day-to-day basis." Other administrators made similar statements. As another administrator at Worldwide colorfully put it, "We are in the protecting our behinds business," alluding to the fact that they had to crosscheck their documentations to ensure they billed correctly for services rendered and kept sound records. Thelma, Rebekah Sankoh's daughter, stated that she frequently told her staff, "If you don't document it, it didn't happen," a mantra other scholars have found among nursing home administrators, as well (Diamond 1992; Rodriquez 2014). Thus, administrators not only had to worry about being personally compliant, but they also had to make sure their staff were properly trained according to the standards set by their funding sources and government policy. For instance, at the end of training and orientation sessions I witnessed at Worldwide and a couple other agencies, attendees had to sign a form acknowledging they had received the training. Miriam found ensuring that paraprofessional nursing staff had all the necessary training for tasks like administering medication to be time consuming and difficult. As she said: "[Medication technicians] have to pass certain tests. You've got to go back and make sure that they are up to speed with how. . . . It's one thing to say that it was done, but it's another thing to prove it. And because we get our license renewed every year, the Department of Health comes and that's [meaning documentation of the training] what they are looking for.

While I observed collegiality between the Johnsons and DC bureaucrats, they, as well as other owners and administrators, felt surveilled and policed by the various departments they engaged with. Jennifer Nazareno (2018) found similar work-related challenges among Filipina owners of home health care businesses and residential care facilities.

At the same time, my observations suggest that the agencies were complying with local and federal regulations and operating ethically. At Worldwide, two sets of meetings stood out to me as exemplars of not only positive patient/provider interactions but also of care that was compliant with local government regulations and in line with industry standards. I observed intake meetings where administrators, usually Malaika, the VP, and the case managers, met with the individuals who had been approved to receive services from their agency. In one instance, Malaika was meeting with Moira Peterson,[10] an older white woman who was scheduled to move into one of the residential care homes. The meeting was held in Malaika's office in the day program. Malaika began by asking Ms. Peterson to write her name and to acknowledge that the information to follow had been read to her. With noticeable patience and kindness, Malaika explained Ms. Peterson's rights as they relate to privacy and other matters. She said that Ms. Peterson had the right to privacy, that people should knock before they entered her room. She also stated that she had the right to "put your stuff in a safe space and get snacks when you want." "You should also have access to all parts of your home," she said. Malaika then went into detail about contact information for relevant household staff should Ms. Peterson encounter any issues or problems. The meeting stood out to me as illustrative of the "person-centered approach" to care that DDS stressed in its policy documents and that agencies like Worldwide tried to instill in their workers.

I also observed the Individual Support Plan, ISP, meetings for a few care recipients. These meetings were used to determine the types and scope of services that should be provided for the individual based on their needs and preferences. They were held annually for every care recipient. The development of the ISPs was a team process in which the individual receiving care, the QIDP ("Q" in the parlance that was popular at Worldwide), house manager, a psychologist or psychiatrist, a social worker, the Services Coordinator at DDS,[11] and the DON or an assigned RN were present. I was told that sometimes family members (parents/legal guardians) of the individual attend, but family members were not present in the cases I observed. The ISP meetings usually took place in the conference room at the day program, but one I witnessed occurred in one of the residential care homes, in this case a small apartment. The apartment was in a condo building and was one of two residences Worldwide operated in the same building. These smaller apartments that were shared by two persons were used to house care recipients who could live somewhat independently. There was Afro-centric art on the wall, and dining chairs and some folding chairs were organized in a circle in the small living room. Miriam chaired the meeting; in addition to me and the care recipient, the house manager for the residence, the QIDP, and six DSPs who serviced the two apartments in the building were in attendance from Worldwide. A psychologist from DDS and the DDS service coordinator also attended, and Kareem, Worldwide's training coordinator, attended by telephone. The Worldwide employees are all West African; the DDS psychologist was a white woman, and the DDS service coordinator was an African American woman.

The care recipient was Ms. Elise Robinson, a forty-five-year-old African American woman, nicely attired in a stylish dress and fashionable flats. She was higher functioning than many of the care receivers I saw, and she engaged actively in conversation with the care staff. Miriam started the meeting by asking Ms. Robinson about her physical health and how she was feeling. Then she went over Ms. Robinson's medical diagnoses and the medications she was taking, including psychotropic medications. She then quizzed the DSPs, who are also trained to administer medications, on why Ms. Robinson was taking specific medications. The short oral quiz was to comply with DDS policy to ensure para-professional staff who administered medications had basic knowledge of the conditions for which they are prescribed. After the quiz, and Miriam seemingly satisfied, the DSPs left the meeting. However, it seems notable that they were there at all. Sociologists Lisa Dodson and Rebekah M. Zincavage (2015), in a study of eighteen long-term care residential facilities in Massachusetts, noted that CNAs were not included in similar meetings about the care concerns of nursing home residents, even though they were at the front lines of care and are supposed to "report" observations of health changes to clinical staff. The fact that the direct care staff who work most intimately with the service recipients were absent from the important deliberations and decision-making about care illustrates the low status of these positions.

The ISP meeting then turned to other aspects of Ms. Robinson's life that were not health related. One goal that was set in a previous ISP was for Ms. Robinson to secure employment. There was then conversation about the ways to make that happen, including enrolling in a work preparedness program and facilitating library visits so she could fill out application forms. Ms. Robinson also shared that she would love to learn to drive, and that was listed as one of her new set of goals. In all, the meeting was positive. Ms. Robinson was consulted in each step and verbally expressed her wishes. While the sequence of events varied, this ISP was similar in format and team composition to the others I witnessed. The main exception was that many other care recipients were nonverbal. In those cases, there was more input from the psychologist/psychiatrists, social workers, and QIDP.

RACIALIZED HIERARCHIES AND "ETHNIC LOGICS" IN AFRICAN-OWNED HEALTH CARE AGENCIES

The interactions between African immigrant entrepreneurs and workers and care recipients like Ms. Robinson was most evident from my observations at Worldwide. In interviews with owners and administrators of other home health and disability support agencies, I asked who made up their staff (including ethnic composition); what attributes they believed they possessed; and how well they did their jobs. Ayo told me that most of his home health aide and nursing staff was West African, although he hired other racial and ethnic groups in professional roles. He said: "I hire two social workers. You know they are high class, they need to go to school, so I have only two, and moreover the Black Americans they do well there, so the social workers that I have they are all Black Americans . . . one of the speech therapists is Spanish [meaning Latinx] and we have two white physical therapists, but the nurses and home health aides, most of them are West Africans."

Ayo's characterizations of his staff by occupational group and race/ethnicity reflect general racialized hierarchies in specializations in skilled medical occupations (Chambliss 1996; George 2005; Yeates 2009). His characterization of some jobs as "high class" illustrates not only the workings of a tiered health care system but also a racial segmentation of the U.S health/long-term care labor market and the "ghettoization" of some segments within the labor sector. Other studies of low-wage, low-prestige care work illuminate racial and gendered segmentation in the care sector and the concentration of immigrant women of color at the bottom of professional hierarchies. In the context of global capitalism, employers, including employers in domestic and low-level care work, ultimately favor a labor force that is deemed "cheap, docile and exploitable." Immigrants, women, and people of color are deemed the most exploitable. Because the native-born largely reject these sectors, care recipients come to prefer immigrants, especially immigrant women of color, in these roles, sometimes attributing effective care to "natural" or cultural characteristics common in particular populations (Chang 2000; Degiuli 2011, 2016; Guevarra 2010; Hondagneu-Sotelo 2001; Parreñas 2001; Rodriguez 2010).

While Ayo had focused on the racial/ethnic composition of his labor force, the Johnsons and Rebekah Sankoh spoke more about their relationships with their majority-West African staff. Rebekah was frustrated with her home care staff's lack of familiarity with U.S. culture and traditions. She described that she often received feedback from care recipients (African American and older white adults) who were dissatisfied with their African care workers. Most of the complaints centered on their inability to make "American foods" like "scrambled eggs," and "they don't know how to do toast," Rebekah reported. For their part, Rebekah and her daughter Thelma told me that aides complained that some clients refused to allow them to keep their home-cooked African meals in their refrigerators "because it's going to stink up [their] food." Rebekah explained these disagreements as personality clashes and the result of demanding clients, but the work of anthropologist Cati Coe (2019) gives us further analytical insight into the nature of these types of interactions. Studying the relationships between African immigrant home care workers and their white care recipients, Coe found that the care workers experienced "racial insults" and humiliations, some of which were centered around food. Care workers felt insulted and humiliated as well as unwelcome when they were asked to eat from different utensils than their employers or, as in this case, were banned from bringing their food into the care recipients' home/space. Even though Rebekah and Thelma did not view these incidents through a racial lens, it is possible that their staff felt similar humiliations and injuries to their sense of self. Despite her claims of "helping" her coethnics through employment, Rebekah, like many of the native-born employers described by Coe, seemed to take the clients' side in these conflicts. To mitigate some of the clients' complaints and dissatisfaction, Rebekah told me she was thinking about incorporating a culinary segment in the trainings she organized for her staff. She had plans to move into a bigger office space, where she said she would simulate a kitchen and train the staff in appropriate American culinary traditions.

The Johnsons did not express frustrations with their staff based on client or family members' complaints. They largely spoke about their assessment of the "fit" and efficiency of West Africans as disability support professionals. For example, Malaika said, "For white Americans and Black Americans, this type of work is not commensurate with their quality-of-life expectations. It is a 24–7, round the clock operation. Even though the money may be good, it does not facilitate the lifestyle of taking vacations, checking out of the office at a decent hour and spending time with family."

Malaika understood that disability support was unattractive for many native-born Americans due, in part, to the long hours, including overnight shifts and the unattractive nature of personal care. She, however, also relied on cultural explanations to explain her largely immigrant workforce. She stated that "the immigrant mentality of work to the bone" or work around the clock encouraged working long hours and tolerating live-in care work rejected by others. She concluded, "It does not conflict with our values in terms of quality of life."

Sociologist Cameron Macdonald identified the role of culture as a tool that employers used to rank and sort employees, especially in childcare, where criteria such as educational credentials—grades, GPA, internships—are not quite as useful as determinants of "fit." She writes, "Employers need ways to sort out and select among different groups of workers beyond criteria used in other markets," education, credentials, experience, etc. Often "employers delve into a 'cultural toolkit; to solve particular life problems" (Macdonald 2015, 154). While drawing from a largely homogenous employee pool, Malaika drew quite explicitly from this cultural toolkit to explain why West Africans were "good at caring." She said: "I just think from a natural perspective, I think is also where the culture component fits in. West Africans just by nature, they are very caring people. We take care of our old. We take care of our young. We can be the most impoverished, but you know, 'if I eat you eat.' [A saying that indicates that they look out for each other]. And that sort of natural spirit comes out during the care that we provide for patients or our residents at the facilities."

My interviews with Malaika and, to a lesser extent her sister Miriam, revealed that they relied on what Macdonald has called "ethnic logics;" that is, "strategies designed to match a certain set of desired services with the presumed characteristics of prospective employees" (Macdonald 2015, 153). Respondents in Macdonald's study used ethnic logics to select workers for specific care needs. For example, midwestern "rural wholesomeness" made for nurturing nannies, or rural Scandinavian nannies were considered better for the infancy stage than cosmopolitan English ones (Macdonald 2010, 2015). Malaika used "ethnic logics" to articulate her personal beliefs about the traits and attributes West Africans possessed, which made them "fit" for the physical as opposed to the intellectual tasks of care. "The African woman is bred to care and nurture. The West African woman in particular is caring and nurturing," she said.

By deploying "ethnic logics," employers like Malaika were, indeed, bringing together "cultural assumptions about the nature of the care to be provided and about the characteristics a worker needs to provide this care" (Macdonald 2015, 154). Malaika's idea that West African workers were good at facilitating the physical and nurturant needs but not the developmental or cognitive needs of their care recipients was like some of the upper middle-class parents described by Macdonald. These employers used ethnic logics to find the "developmentally ideal nanny;" that is, the nanny who they believed had the right characteristics and traits to facilitate the cognitive and developmental ability of their children at older ages. They contrasted the "developmentally ideal" nanny to the nurturant nanny who was ideal for the comforting and caring tasks for infants and toddlers. They cast young European au-pairs or Midwestern white nannies as the developmentally ideal nanny, in contrast to older immigrant Black Caribbean nannies or Spanish-speaking nannies from specific national groups being better suited to nurturing. The fact that the Johnsons used similar ethnic logics to those Macdonald found among American parents suggests that they understood and had a facility with U.S. racial/ethnic formations and stereotypes. They also were savvy in marketing their employees utilizing ethnic logics often found to be used by other employers in nurturant care work (Degiuli 2016; Guevarra 2010; Parreñas 2001). The apparent dissatisfaction with their African staff's intellectual, developmental, and cognitive care work also points to the lack of competition for these jobs.

Cameron Macdonald stressed ethnicity as opposed to a central focus on race and other social statuses. I find the concept of ethnic logics useful for my analysis of employers and employees with a shared ethnicity and in a single geographic location. In fact, the Johnsons referenced culture/ethnicity, and to a lesser extent gender, rather than other social statuses such as race when describing recruitment strategies and employee relations. But other studies of care work have suggested that gendered and racialized logics are foundational to the ways in which employer's make judgments about workers' suitability for specific tasks of care (Colen 1989, 1991; Degiuli 2016; Glenn 2010; Guevarra 2010; Liang 2011; Parreñas 2001; Rollins 1985; Yeates 2009). Racialized and gendered logics inform the "cultural toolkit" from which employers make their judgments and assess "fit" among diverse racial/ethnic groups. Race and gender also are central to *how* hierarchies are created among different racial/ethnic/national groups. As sociologist Francesca Degiuli concluded from her study of Italian employers of elder care workers: "Employers use stereotypes, preconceived notions about race and ethnicity, anecdotal experience, and hearsay to find help needed in the shortest amount of time, creating and reproducing stigmatizing hierarchies very difficult for immigrant workers to escape. . . . These hierarchies in turn affect which women will get the best jobs and which will get the most demanding and less remunerative ones" (Degiuli 2016, 86–87).

Adding an interrogation of racialized and gendered ideologies to Cameron's conceptualization of ethnic logics allows us to see how this sort of sorting, ranking, and rationalization of fit through the lens of culture inheres globally and in multiple locations, with preferences and hierarchies taking peculiar forms in distinct contexts at various times. For instance, perceptions of Filipinas as preferred care workers in Italy, or in Rhacel Parreñas' terms, the "Mercedes Benz of care workers" compared to Black or Latinx groups (Parreñas 2001, 178). Francesca Degiuli (2016) found that Italian employers of elder care workers tended to prefer Peruvians and Filipinos over Albanians and Africans. In other studies, Southeast Asian immigrant women care workers have frequently been ascribed essential characteristics by employers; for example, perceived as having a natural inclination to care for others, as well as being docile and controllable, traits "which employers attribute to cultures with a strong work ethic and values related to family, loyalty, and authority" (Guevarra 2010, 10). They have thus been viewed by recruiters, the nation state, and some employers in Asian contexts as "ideal maids" (Liang 2011), or the "ideal migrant subject" (Rodriguez and Schewenken 2013). Conceptions of Black Caribbean nannies, on the other hand, have shifted over time from being "ideal nannies" to being "loud and difficult" or "uneducated island girls" (Guevarra 2010). While not expressing a racialized preference, Ayo Adebayo's characterizations of African American and Latinx social workers as "high class" compared to West African home care aides fit within this long history of racialized, gendered, and ethnic logics in care hierarchies.

For the Johnson family, ethnic logics were not used to screen and sort or create hierarchies among various racial/ethnic groups, because most of the labor supply were Africans, often from the same national group, with very little competition from outsiders. They used ethnic logics to rationalize the fit of Africans for the direct, hands-on care; in other words, the "dirty work" of care. The Johnsons also used ethnic logics to criticize those coethnic employees who in their view did not meet specific ethical, bureaucratic, intellectual, and professional standards/goals set by the agency and the DC disability support establishment, including to develop cognitive and developmental ability. Those employees were "not good at facilitating the personhood" of care recipients, according to Malaika. There was a major irony, however, in that the Johnsons' characterization of West Africans as "natural" direct care workers was at odds with the experiences of their staff. As I will describe in more detail in the following chapter, staff found the work of caring far from "natural."

4 · DISABILITY SUPPORT
The Transformation of Immigrants into Care Workers

I arrived at the day program for adults with disabilities run by Worldwide around 10 o'clock on a Monday morning, just in time to witness the arrival of the first group of program attendees. They arrived in the company of residential staff from group homes run by Worldwide or other agencies. All were adults; many appeared to be in their thirties and forties, though a few were older. Most had backpacks, and some also carried lunch boxes. All care recipients and all the staff were Black. Clients were African American, and staff were West African. While this was the demographic I observed on this day, on other occasions I noticed a few white care recipients. The care recipients all exhibited observable physical and developmental disabilities. At other times, I noticed that some care recipients used adaptive equipment like walking sticks or walkers, and some were in wheelchairs. A few wore helmets. Residential staff filled out a sign-in sheet at the front desk, indicating each client's name, time of drop off, and the caregiver's initials. Sometimes the residential staff literally handed the client off to the day program support staff, who held severely disabled care recipients' hands and walked with them to rooms at the back of the building. The residential staff were wearing plain clothes, while the day program staff all wore t-shirts with the name of the agency emblazoned on them.

The individuals were sorted into groups of eight to ten people in classrooms the agency called group homes. Each was named for a neighborhood in Washington, DC; for example, Capitol Hill, Fort Totten, Adams Morgan, Logan, Georgia-Pentworth, and Foggy Bottom. Each room had two or three direct support professionals, who were referred to as counselors within that setting, with one designated the lead counselor. One of the classrooms had huge posters on the walls depicting wildfires, tornadoes, and other forms of natural disasters. Another classroom had tools for artwork set up on the work desks. On those walls were posters of a few U.S presidents, and on one end were posters depicting numbers in large font. There was a world map mounted on the other end of the room. A third classroom also had pictures depicting various natural disasters, alongside safety signs and dates/calendar posters. The final classroom I observed was set up with a big television screen, and I noticed a video game console positioned nearby.

Care recipients were sorted based on their intellectual and cognitive abilities and skillsets, and there appeared to be more female care recipients than males. The male caregivers all were assigned to the all-male rooms. Some groups were doing art therapy; I noticed one group making items using popsicle sticks. Another group was playing board games. Another had group members listening to peaceful meditation music while others were sitting quietly. As Miriam, the director of nursing, walked by, several of the individuals receiving care addressed her by her first name. She engaged warmly with care recipients and addressed them as Mr. or Ms. and their first names. As I engaged Miriam in conversation in the hallway, a client, an older woman, approached and hugged her, and then me. Another client, a younger man, gave us an enthusiastic high five.

Witnessing these overall positive and respectful interactions led me to ponder the relations of care developed between middle-class West African immigrant care workers (many of whom came from non-health care backgrounds), and a mostly low-income, older, African American care clientele. How did these migrants make sense of their role in care occupations, especially working with severely intellectually and physically disabled persons? What role did the agencies play in creating these workers? How did class status and professional experience prior to migration shape the identities they later developed? Were there gendered differences between men and women? In what ways did experiences in disability support transform immigrant DSPs, and how did these transformations shape their interactions and relationships with clients? What are the implications for our understanding of migrant labor within care occupations?

Unlike some workers in higher-status care positions, such as nurses, prior to migration, many DSPs had little exposure to institutionalized or long-term care for people with severe physical and intellectual disabilities. Like many others in the study, some got into the field because care pioneers, (family, friends, and/or acquaintances) introduced them to paid care work when they arrived in the United States. Many started working without a clear working knowledge of disability support. For example, Joy Etoundie, who had been a high school math and science teacher in Cameroon, joined a care pioneer, in this case a friend, in applying for a job as a DSP at a Cameroonian-owned agency soon after arriving in the United States. Joy recalled: "I didn't even know what DSP was." Her friend told her what the DSP acronym referred to, but when she asked for further details, the friend told her she only needed to fill out the application form properly. As it happened, Joy did not have to wait to hear from the placement agency, as she explained: "[A different friend] just turned and told me, 'You've got a job.'

I said, 'What?' She said, 'This lady [a private individual not connected to any agency] is calling me saying that the mother needs help.' I asked, 'Who is going to orientate me on this?' She said, 'It's simple, it's just simple helping somebody in the house to cook and things like that.' That's how, two weeks after I got here [to the United States], I got that job."

The experience of being thrust into the field shortly after arriving in the United States was common among some immigrant care workers like Joy. Care pioneers with longer tenure in the United States, keen to initiate their newly arrived friends and relatives into care work, presented providing care in clients' homes as natural and simple. Immigrants like Joy, who initially found work in the informal "gray market" for elder care—that is, home care jobs offered and negotiated privately with family members—later found their jobs to be far from simple. As Joy explained, her lack of familiarity with basic medical assistive devices and equipment proved a complication. For example, she described an incident while putting a client to bed: "When I put her [client] on the bed, then she asked me to bring the commode, I had never seen a commode in my life. I said, 'What is it?' She said, 'That thing.' It dawned on me, that, oh, I see people come to America and clean [referencing bowel movements, but using language that may be offensive to reader], so this is it.'" As this comment implied, for some respondents, it was only after they had started work that they began to make sense of care work or to associate direct care work with performing unpleasant tasks.

Institutional care facilities like Worldwide and state-funded home care agencies provided training and orientation for new DSPs and followed the strict protocols established by the Washington, DC, Department of Disability Services, but many care workers still felt unprepared for their roles at first. A case manager at Worldwide recalled his first day on the job when he was a DSP: "I'd gone through orientation, and they got me ready for what was going on. But it wasn't any close to what I actually did that first day. I guess I was a rookie, all right."

When I sat in on job interviews and attended orientation sessions with new staff members at Worldwide, I found that administrators focused most of their attention on detailing the policies that govern work with this population of care recipients. For example, they told new employees how to document the care that was received using agency-provided worksheets (for billing and assessment purposes) and went over emergency procedures such as fire evacuations plans, etc. A one-on-one training I observed included a description of the chain of command at Worldwide, information regarding the new employee's direct supervisors, and the protocols to follow if he observed "serious reportable incidents" such as neglect, exploitation, signs of illness, bruises on a patient, falls, or accidents. Other topics tangentially referenced care but did not address what to expect in terms of actual physical contact and interactions with clients or how to deal with one's own emotions on the job.[1] In this training, the solo orientee was educated on what was termed the "Persons First Language Policy." Through this policy, the agency stressed the use of appropriate and humanizing language. They encouraged disability support professionals to address care recipients by their given names, never to use pejorative terms, and to use "the persons we serve," when referencing them in the third person. Workers also were told they should not use "mental retardation" but "intellectual disability." The only further guidance as to how to interact with clients were statements like, "Treat them [care recipients] like you would treat your family member." Here, the staff trainer paused. With a wry smile, he continued: "Well, a family member that you really like." I noticed that a few employees who had completed training still had no idea what their day-to-day duties would be, and in the case of the young man mentioned above, did not even know what their job title would be.

Augustine Marah, a Sierra Leonean immigrant who, like Joy, taught science and math prior to migration, said he had not had prior contact with people with intellectual disabilities and was unfamiliar with the behaviors associated with this population of care recipients when he first started out. Describing his first care recipient in a group home, he stated: "He was really a difficult person. That was my first time in the field. I did not know much." Due to their general unfamiliarity with formalized care of individuals with intellectual and physical disabilities, many immigrants I met struggled when they started work. Many recalled feelings of shock on their first day on the job.

Describing his first day on the job, Nelson Sandy, a Sierra Leonean Qualified Intellectual Disability Professional working with Worldwide said:

So, I start there [at the day program] and I get there my first day I sit there. I'm actually reading the Behavioral Support Plan and everything. It doesn't tell me a lot about their [the clients'] behaviors, who has what. The second day, the lead counselor . . . does not show up. So, I'm there, literally, by myself. Secondly, that's the time I found out one of the people's behaviors is that they smear feces on themselves. . . . No worry, but when I take him to the bathroom, I find out that he has a prolapse. At this point, I am disgusted. There is poop everywhere in the bathroom. I'm cleaning and I'm telling myself, "If I come here tomorrow, if I go home and I come here tomorrow, I'm going to be at this job for a long time."

Many DSPs mentioned that they thought about leaving the field after the first day, but just like Nelson, not only did they stay but the impulse to leave lessened over time. Musu Fofana, another Sierra Leonean, who now worked as a house manager but started out as DSP, recalled: "It was that day when I started, I was supposed to go with [my client] as a one-on-one [direct support to a physically disabled client] to his day program. He had all kinds of behavioral issues. He was somebody that would eat just inedibles. And he will, you know, like, elope [wander off]. And I called my mom. I was like, 'After today I'm not coming back.' It was so funny, my mom said to me, 'Well, just do it for a week and see what you think.'"

Musu took her mother's advice and did decide to stay.

Other respondents also had memories, like Nelson's, of being unceremoniously left alone to provide care in their early days in the field. Aspects of personal care, especially cleaning bowel movements and bathing patients, could be quite distressing. Nurse Y,[2] one of the nurses who administered medications and provided other routine health care for the individuals in the day program recalled her early experiences as a direct support professional. She recalled, "taking care of the individuals, the things I had never done before [was difficult]. It was so hard for me to see them, cleaning them when they use the bathroom. Sometimes it was hard for me to even eat after I had been cleaning them, so after three months of that, I said I can't do this anymore, so I stopped [working as a DSP]." She later returned to health care after training to be a nurse.

DSPs from middle-class backgrounds prior to migration found their entry into low-status health care work particularly distressing. Michaela Johnson-Smith was a middle-aged Sierra Leonean house manager for one of the residential homes operated by Worldwide when we spoke, but she had entered the field as a DSP. Fashionably dressed, with perfectly coiffed hair and professional-looking makeup, Michaela told me her story as we sat at the dining table in one of the homes managed by Worldwide. I watched her becoming increasingly distressed as she described her first days as a DSP. Michaela had been an administrative assistant for an international aid organization in Sierra Leone. Her husband held a high position in the Sierra Leonean military, and she said she lived a comfortable and pampered life before they emigrated. She and her husband made the decision to move to the United States because they believed he would get better treatment for a medical condition. She described her first experiences at her first job in the United States as a DSP: "To be honest with you, this job, when I started working, when it's time to come to work, I will cry like a baby. I would cry. I will weep as if they said, oh your mother just passed away. [In many parts of Sierra Leone, it is understood that 'a mother's death' refers to the greatest sorrow.] When you think where you were [in terms of class status before emigration] and then come to this new set up. I was like, oh my God. I will never forget the very first day of work."

References to persistent tears were not uncommon. The pain that previously middle-class subjects felt because of their status loss was palpable. In addition to coping with the physical demands of the work, many struggled emotionally with the fact that they were literally performing "dirty work."

While they initially found some of their care duties distressing, research subjects could simultaneously earn incomes that could not only sustain them in the United States but also allow them to send valuable remittances home. According to the U.S. Bureau of Labor Statistics,[3] in 2018, the median annual wage of personal care aides working in service provision for the elderly and persons with disabilities was $24,060. However, respondents also worked overtime shifts, which usually paid higher hourly rates, or combined two or more part-time care jobs with different employers to augment pay rates. Mobility within Worldwide and elsewhere in the industry also guaranteed a concomitant increase in wages. DSPs had every hope of attaining positions as qualified intellectual disability professionals, which meant they might earn, on average, $54,000. House managers/case managers like Michaela, responsible for supervising the paraprofessional staff in the residential homes operated by the company or administrative tasks at the day program, earned a yearly salary of $47,000. The company administrators told me that, on average, current DSPs had been employed with Worldwide for two or more years, QIDPs and other mid-level staff for an average of over five years, and senior management for over ten years, showing that working in immigrant-owned spaces provided job security for workers in a marginalized occupation. Working in private homes or group homes also allowed some live-in DSPs to save on housing costs and provided flexibility to study for other licensures in health care. The fact that the work was generally low status but provided flexibility and the opportunity to augment income or gain professional mobility within the company created a sense of what I have termed class ambivalence among research participants.

The concept of "contradictory class mobility," which sociologist Rhacel Parreñas (2001, 2015) identified among Filipino domestic workers in Rome and Los Angeles applied to study participants who had been middle-class in their home countries but found themselves in low-status work in the United States. Parreñas described how middle-class Filipinas coped with their realities as lower-status domestics while simultaneously earning significantly higher incomes than they had in the Philippines. Parreñas highlighted the contradiction in their experiences in financial terms, as while working as domestics in the global north, they were able to afford to hire domestics for their own childcare needs. The fact that high-status workers in the global south can earn less than their low-status counterparts in the global north thus captures the unequal positioning of countries in the global economy. To cope with the class dislocations they encountered, middle-class Filipinas, according to Parreñas, activated four major strategies. First, they performed domestic work "under the fantasy of reversal;" that is, they dreamed of returning to the Philippines where they would be served by their own domestic servants. These fantasies of reversal enabled them to tolerate the routine indignities they encountered as domestics in Rome and Los Angeles. Second, they downplayed the decline in their social status by emphasizing the higher racial status employers granted them in comparison to their Black and Latina domestic counterparts. Third, some domestics tried to resolve the contradictions in their class status by embracing closeness and intimacy with their employers; for instance, by embracing narratives that cast them as "one of the family" rather than domestic servants. Finally, some domestics embraced "deference and maternalism." In other words, they embraced subservience to extract higher gains from their employers.

Similarly, by class ambivalence, I articulate the process where West African immigrants had to adapt to the loss of premigration occupational prestige, renegotiate their class positions, and enact strategies to manage their identities and find dignity and meaning in their new professional lives. However, class ambivalence goes beyond class contradictions shaped by disparities in earnings due to the unequal location of countries within the global political economy. In fact, many in disability support were reluctant to provide details about their earnings in the United States, or to frame their experiences within the prism of financial gain or loss. Class ambivalence describes the subjective and psychological states of ambivalence that developed among disability support professionals who had the opportunity to work in an environment controlled by coethnics and the prospect of mobility at the company or within the industry, but simultaneously had to perform care tasks they found demeaning, degrading, and distressing, often for lower-class recipients. This process of adjusting to their new social and professional lives in America often led to a reassessment of the benefits of migration against the costs of status loss.

When I asked Michaela, the Sierra Leonean house manager mentioned earlier, about whether the reality of life in the United States had matched her premigration expectations, she said:

> You know back home, this first world, people are so crazy [i.e., eager] to come here. I will never forget, when I was about to come here when I bid goodbye to my friends back home at a send-off party they had for me, all of them were so excited that I was leaving, and they said that America is six miles to heaven. But when I came here, I met someone who I knew from back home and she told me welcome to six miles to hell [laughing]. Those people back home they think its heaven, here they think it's hell.

"What about you? What do you think?" I asked her, and she said, simply, "Purgatory . . . between hell and heaven." Her word choice captures the sense of a between state. On the one hand, DSPs suffered from the loss of status and downward occupational mobility associated with care work. On the other hand, they could earn money that provided for themselves and their family members back home, and some would be able to fund further credentials to advance their careers in health care. They also worked in institutions dominated by members of their ethnic/national groups. These institutions also provided some autonomy and the potential for increased professional responsibility.

Amos Ngo, a manager of a health care recruitment agency who had been an aeronautic engineer in Cameroon, experienced class ambivalence. I spoke with

him in the small reception room of the agency where he staffed the front desk—
received staff, job applicants, and visitors to the agency, and answered the telephone. Amos got increasingly agitated as he recalled several instances in his past
where he felt disparaged and demeaned by clients. He said:

> When you go to work with them [care recipients] they have the impression that
> you are so desperate. You are second-class. I mean, I'm working with somebody
> who cannot write his name, and he is looking down at me. I tell him, "Look. I am
> a seasoned—I've been to school. The schools I've been to, you'll never be there."
> It got to a point where one day I went home, I brought my pictures when I'm in
> the aircraft, in uniform, to the camera [looking into the camera]. I say [to care
> recipient], "You don't talk to me now because I'm no riffraff. You don't talk." I
> said, "Don't think I'm here because I like it. I'm here because I have to work." And
> the guy looked at me. So that makes the job where . . . where somebody looks at
> you as if you're inferior or whatever. . . . it's really sometimes annoying, degrad-
> ing. The way they ask, the way they talk to you.

In addition to dealing with his status loss, Amos took great offence at being
bossed around and treated with perceived disrespect: "You come to work with
somebody who tells you, 'You've got to stay outside. Wait outside for some time.'
Even the last client I had before I said I don't want to work in this field anymore
[recalling the last client before he left direct care work], I come to this lady's
house in the morning. She would keep me outside in the lobby till maybe 11:00.
She says she's sleeping. 'I don't want a disturbance.' 'So, can I go home?' 'No, you
don't have to go. I need you.' . . . She gets up."

As Amos described his duties, he highlighted the feminized nature of the
work: "Now I start maybe cleaning her house, take her dresses to laundry. You
know, work for a woman. There are things for a woman. . . . Look, there are
things that, back in Africa, I can't do. You see a lady who will take her underwears
and tell you to go wash them in—down here, they wash them in machines. So, I
put on gloves. I do the job."

Amos's interactions with clients with physical disabilities and other chronic
conditions as described above were different from the others, who worked with
clients with intellectual disabilities. The care workers who worked with individuals with intellectual disabilities did not mention being made to feel inferior by
their clients, nor did they exhibit feelings of anger and hostility such as Amos
expressed. However almost all the workers in disability support felt diminished
by having to perform tasks like bathing, cleaning, and washing intimate effects.
They felt pain at the loss of their professional status and class privilege, but some
stressed, as Amos did, that they coped with the negative feelings simply because
they needed work and had few alternatives.

Amos's experience and that of others I met illustrate what sociologist Cynthia Cranford has described as the "complex power dynamic between recipients and workers who encounter different axes of oppression" (Cranford 2020, 11). Here, Amos, a Black African immigrant male, able-bodied, and class-privileged from the point of view of his premigration educational and professional status, was resentful of the downward occupational and professional mobility he had encountered after migration. His resentment seemed to be heightened because of his perceived mistreatment by care recipients who themselves experienced multiple layers of disadvantage. Recall his perception of being looked down upon by uneducated care recipients "who can't even write [their] name." His description of his interactions with one care recipient, a Black native-born American physically disabled woman, lesser educated and a recipient of state-subsidized care, who treated him with disdain and disrespect crystallized these complex intersections of power, privilege, and simultaneous disadvantage and disempowerment. Some studies that have focused on the relational dynamics between care workers and care recipients with physical disabilities show that care recipients value "respectful negotiations over what is done when, where and how it is done" (Cranford 2020, 10). They also seek autonomy, control, the ability to communicate their needs effectively, and to trust new carers in their home to provide physical assistance in ways they perceive as secure. At the same time, these needs can be misinterpreted and misunderstood by care workers and lead to conflict (Gibson et al. 2007 Meyer et al. 2007; Twigg 1999, 2000; Ungerson 1999). I don't have enough information to assess the care recipients' actions in this case. However, overall, Amos's account of fraught encounters and negative emotional responses was mediated by intra-racial classed and gendered struggles between himself and care recipients also marginalized by their race, class, gender, and disability.

The affront to masculinity and the resulting loss of dignity was common among male care workers and reflected rather dramatically in Amos's resentment at having to wash a female client's underwear. To recoup some of his dignity, Amos went out of his way to assert his professional identity and to reframe his relationship with his care recipients as a professional working one rather than one of servitude. He reported that he often told clients: "'I came to help you, not you helping me. Because that's it. I will work with you. I don't work for you. I work for an agency, but I work with you, because you are a client.' That idea, see? 'I am a staff in an agency, and we work together. So, I work with you. I don't work for you.'"

Amos's professional posture as an employee who worked through an "agency," as opposed to being a "maid" in private employment, reflects the gendered implications of direct care work as paid employment and the historical continuity between paid reproductive care work and domestic service (Coe 2019; Duffy 2005, 2007). Other male participants expressed general discomfort with caring for female care recipients and performing intimate care labor. Augustine told me that he had considered becoming a registered nurse but did not pursue nursing because he felt uncomfortable providing intimate care (bathing, cleaning) for female patients. Worldwide allowed him to work closely and intimately with only male care recipients, even if it meant remaining at the status and salary level of a QIDP instead of a nurse. Another group of care workers that expressed similar concerns were young women registered nurses. A few reported that they felt deeply uncomfortable to be asked to provide intimate care for male care recipients when they worked as direct care workers. One registered nurse was so distressed and bothered about being exposed to male nudity, she told me, that she cried often.

In contrast to some women who admitted to crying on the job, Amos, the disgruntled DSP, described maintaining a pleasant disposition as another tool to maintain his dignity: "I [wash my female client's underwear] the way she wants with a smiling face, because when you start looking at your own self with pity, you know you've lost it. So, I do it as if I enjoy the job, because after they've paid my money, I need the money. I do the job. I do the job. Every day, I have to come clean up the place. They treat me like a maid. That is the most degrading part."

He was unusual in performing emotional labor by "smiling" and maintaining a pleasant disposition to cope with feminized caring labor. Male care workers often utilized what I term "discourses of need" or "survival." They said they did care work because they needed to work and survive and could not continue in premigration occupations. They thus articulated a form of masculinity that centered their hard work and dedication and the idea that they "would do anything" to survive. They also used these 'discourses of need" or "survival" to offset the impact of doing work that was not traditionally associated with hegemonic masculinity. Amos, who had used his experience in direct care to become a manager at a higher salary, described the calculation made by many: "By the time you have money [from DSP work], you can pay for another course, another course that is professionally better than what you're doing. You now move. Maybe you do CNA or maybe something good, start real nursing. While you go to school, you're working."

Viewing work as a DSP as a steppingstone that would enable him to move into a better paying job in health care, Amos also was presenting himself as an ambitious and calculated actor, thus reinterpreting his actions within the toolkit of traditional masculinity.

Utilizing "discourses of need," Adewumi Johnson, a Sierra Leonean DSP who had taken on a second job providing in-home care for a client he described as difficult, said that he had prayed: "Well, God, you know that I have left my kids in Africa and I surely really need this [second] job, because I cannot really rely on [my job at Worldwide]. So, go out here with me. I hear this person I'm going to work with is very difficult; go ahead with me and show me what I'm going to do."

Similarly, Albert Kamara, a QIDP who had been a university lecturer in Sierra Leone, mentioned that he gave up his dreams of working as an economist after he migrated to the United States and became aware of discrimination in the labor market. Health care, at least, he reasoned, would allow him to "put bread and butter on the table." In line with past studies of how men reaffirm their masculinities in female dominated occupations (Cottingham, 2013; Williams, 1991; Wingfield 2009; Scrinzi 2010), the men at Worldwide made sense of their continued location in a feminized field by stressing their breadwinning role and/or applying discourses of survival or need. In that way, research participants made "women's work" compatible with their masculine roles of provider and breadwinner. A few women participants who were single parents also used discourses of need and survival, which they tended to frame as needing to provide for or "feed" their children. Thus, there were slight gender differences between men and women; for example, more men used discourses of need compared to women, and single mothers were the women more likely to use discourses of need, reflecting their material reality as sole providers and breadwinners for their families. Men and women, however, had largely similar experiences of downward mobility and labor market displacement upon migration. Similarly, in a study of well-educated, middle-class, largely English-speaking African immigrants in Vancouver, Canada, sociologist Gillian Creese found that both men and women took entry-level, low-status jobs, which she termed "survival jobs," after migrating to Canada and experiencing "deskilling." As one of her participants put it, "I have to do any type of job in order to survive" (Creese 2011, 83).

While the male respondents in this study were more likely to use discourses of need and survival in addressing their entry and tenure in disability support and to stress their breadwinning roles, both men and women drew from their class backgrounds or previous occupational status and experiences to cope with their new professional lives. This was in marked contrast to the domestics in Parreñas's (2001, 2015) study who regretted that domestic work did not allow them to use their previous skills and made them "stupid." Amos said of his early years as a DSP: "All my [adult] life, for eighteen years, I'd been working on airplanes, but now I was in a different field, caring for people, and people, when you see their conditions, they are really bad. Out of compassion, you have to move for them, work for them, and you are paid something, you know? Now, I've been working with one, two, three, and four clients. They give me a worldwide experience."

Going from working mostly with technology and machinery to a situation dealing intimately with people involved significant emotional labor. Amos highlighted the new skills he had learned as a result, and believed that, despite initial difficulties, disability support taught him compassion and empathy, attributes he seemed to value.

Other immigrants who had previous experiences in service-oriented and people-centered fields drew from the skills and experiences they already possessed. They made meaning by not only drawing from professional experience from their home country but also non-health care jobs they had held after migration. For example, two men who had worked in the hospitality industry after migrating to the United States used the language of customer service and applied their experiences dealing with clients in the hotel industry to their work dealing with clients in disability support. Roland Mason, a Sierra Leonean case manager at Worldwide, stated: "I had worked in the hotel industry where you're dealing with extremely rich people day in, day out. It was the opposite spectrum for me [working at Worldwide], and I actually happened to like [disability support] better cause this will really tell you what's making a difference. There you're doing everything, moving heaven and earth for them, and there was no appreciation at all. They thought giving you money will make everything okay, but here it's just that human factor, basically just helping somebody live their life. I thought that was just the most fruitful thing ever."

Another Sierra Leonean case manager at Worldwide, Sheikh Diallo, said: "I didn't seem to have a problem with [care recipients] because, again, my background was hospitality. It was service . . . the product is just a different product. We're dealing with paying customers in the hotel; now you're dealing with individuals who are the persons that we serve. It was a no-brainer, plus you were doing something that you are capable of doing for people that can't do for themselves. I had no issue with that. It almost came natural for me."

Both Roland and Sheikh felt care recipients were more deserving than the wealthy and privileged clients they had served in the elite segment of the hospitality industry. Therefore, they felt that the services they offered in disability support were more meaningful as they helped to better the human condition.

DSPs who had been teachers in the home country also felt they could draw on past work experiences. They viewed their role as caregivers for people with intellectual disabilities as applying the same principles of education they had applied to their neurotypical students in their past lives. They reinterpreted their role in care work as teaching individuals with varying levels of capability the tools that would make them healthy and productive, both intellectually and physically. As Joy said: "Back home, I used to be a Sunday school teacher. Actually, the only people I have not worked with were the old, because I have worked with children in Sunday school, and I worked with teenagers in school and in high school, and I know how to teach a lot."

Anwar Sheriff, a Sierra Leonean administrator at a home care agency, summarized the views of care workers who believed that past professional experiences had helped them survive in disability support: "[Agency] has a lot of clients to serve, and believe me, I like what we're doing for the people. Basically, I like serving people. I've seen myself in that situation for all of this time, being in the field of teaching, working in the hotel industry, coming over here, working in group homes and stuff, so it's all about people right now." Here, Anwar believed that his mission was to serve people and he drew from the experiences he had amassed through the years.

Albert, a care worker mentioned earlier, utilized a different strategy to cope with his move from being a middle-class professional and part of the intelligentsia in Sierra Leone to working as a disability support professional. While he had achieved educational and professional success as a university professor prior to migration, he drew on his humble background in rural Sierra Leone to explain his approach to his caregiving roles. Explaining how he adapted to care work, he stated:

> For me it was not that stressful, because I had a very humble beginning. [Being a DSP] was not far from my life growing up as a boy. I was a shepherd boy, so helping people was like, [when I was a professor] I was lecturing people with a higher level of IQ but now I am helping people with developmental disability. For me, it was not very far from what I was used to do growing up as a little boy. So, when I came to help others, I was so much into it that there came a time, I loved it. I didn't even look further to say I wanted a job as an economist or policy analyst. . . . The way you can survive if you came from a higher level in life, like from being a lecturer to this field, your background growing up helps you a lot. If you have a background where you had a silver spoon in your mouth, and now you are coming to adapt to a lifestyle which is not silver spoon per se, you are going to face reality and you are going to find it difficult. I had a very humble background, where I had reared and taken care of goats, sheep, cows. So, for me it was okay. I have seen lot of staff come, they can't hold on for a month, they will leave. It depends on the person. Your background will help you a lot to be in this field.

Like other teachers, Albert drew meaning from his current interactions with his clients and interpreted his role as teaching them the life skills and tools they needed to survive. However, by framing his current experiences in disability support within the context of his impoverished upbringing, he drew a parallel between himself and other workers from more privileged backgrounds like Amos, Michaela, Nelson, and Musu. He continued by saying:

> If you don't have a humble background, then you're not going to make it. Or you've not seen the worst part of life. When I was in Sierra Leone, the war in Sierra Leone, I saw a lot of difficult lives, and I also lived that life, so coming [to the United States], it was like a plus for me. With all the amenities that are here in the US and then working with people [with intellectual disabilities] whom I am able to help and transform. So, I was happy seeing them, going out with them, community outings. And they would come back, they are happy. We interact. So,

for me, my life was okay. I do not find it stressful to transition from being a lecturer to DSP.

Other care workers made similar claims, that having gone through challenging life circumstances and/or possessing positive character traits of humility and perseverance in the face of adversity helped some workers cope better than others. Augustine represented this group in this statement:

I am somebody that nothing can really . . . how can I put this? I am really, like, open to change. There's nothing I can really say, I'm too good for this [to do]. Because if you say you are good for certain stuff you are not the right person for this field, because you have to do cleaning, taking the person to the bathroom . . . you clean, you change. That was a very new experience for me, but I got used to it, that was not like a big deal for me. I did not really like struggle with it.

Similarly, Carole Thomas, a Sierra Leonean QIDP, said: "When you enter this field you have to forget that you have an undergraduate degree [earned from home], you have to do what you have to do. It humbles you." Sheikh also felt he had traits that helped him be successful. As he said: "I'm a people person. I'm a caring person. Most people, I've seen over the years, some people come, they're almost scared to death. 'Oh, my goodness, is this what I have to do?'"

Sheikh's words introduce what sociologist Clare Stacey has characterized as the "caring self"—a unique persona or coping strategy that care workers possess or develop because of their work. Some West African disability support professionals reiterated this theme of a caring self as a characteristic some care workers possessed. Roland, the case manager, also stated: "My first day was very interesting. But, like I said, it's just one of those things when you start your first day, you either gonna like it or you don't." Miriam, the DON at Worldwide, said of disability support: "Unfortunately, it's not the type of job you can just do if you really genuinely don't have an interest in it. And sometimes your interest, even though it's not something that you intentionally planned, you fall into it, and genuinely love it." As these words indicate, some people cultivated a "caring self" that they believed helped them excel in their work as care providers for intellectually and physically disabled persons. Many noted that, while initially unfamiliar with the field or reluctant to enter it, they found themselves transformed as they developed new attitudes toward care. While many viewed caring as an intrinsic quality that some people possessed, a few respondents seemed to realize that caring was a skill that could be developed, or at the very least a flexible set of traits and attributes that could be developed and deployed to match varying circumstances. Reflecting this attitude, Miriam stated that she thought having the "personality" the job required and being "flexible" were very important. "Something happens every single day," she said. "Even today, I'm supposed to meet with you, somebody had a fall. I got that call at midnight. And it just changes how your day goes the next day. You know what I mean?"

Administrators and owners of care businesses also described their ideal care workers as possessing traits that could be characterized as a "caring self." Princess Bockarie, a senior administrator at Worldwide, explained a difference she perceived between workers who possessed a caring self and others who didn't: "So, have we had people who, this did not work for them? Absolutely. But a majority, I mean, if you have just the fundamental caring spirit, it's not difficult. You get attached to [patients] if anything." Some comments aligned with sociologist Everett Hughes's finding that imbuing work with Christian values can make "dirty" work "tolerable, or even glorious" (Hughes 1994, 61). Although none of the participants in disability support made direct references to religion, they did invoke spiritual language to make sense of their work and to gain dignity and meaning in work tasks. For example, Joy said of her return to disability support after leaving for a brief stint in IT: "I believe it's a calling because this job is not paying me as much as the IT job will pay me. I came back. I just came back to healthcare again. I believe it's just a calling." Albert described a transformation that occurred shortly after he started working as DSP in explicit spiritual language. He said: "The first experience as a DSP, I was a novice to the field. But I came to realize that helping others was a divine outcome. It was very divine. I did not know, after two weeks of training, things did not sink in well, but with time, most of the areas that were discussed in the two-week training, I was able to understand them. And then I plan myself."

TRANSFORMATION OF MIGRANTS INTO CARE WORKERS

Musu, the Sierra Leonean DSP whose mother convinced her to stick it out a week when she wanted to quit after the first day, said: "At the end of the week, I was in love [with the clients]. I'm like, I'm not going anywhere. And I'm going to stay and see what I can do [to help the people here]." Just like Musu, almost all the disability support professionals I got to know at Worldwide described a transformational process as they developed feelings of empathy and affection for the people for whom they cared. Musu explained the patterns and transformations she had seen in her work over the years:

> I believe that a lot of the way we interact with these people that we serve, makes a big difference in [their lives]. It really does. Because I believe that once they are confident that you care about their wellbeing . . . I mean, they're going to have behaviors because that's who they are. But it's not like we cannot manage, the behaviors. It's that we care enough about them. . . . Like, this guy I was telling you about, he had all kinds of [difficult] behaviors. He doesn't exhibit that anymore. I've been with him for like seven years. He doesn't exhibit that anymore. It amazes me. The other guy . . . [he'll] get into all kinds of trouble. When I started in that home, that guy would not take showers for like weeks. Now he takes a shower almost every day. You know, he works with everybody. So, we've come a long way.

In addition to personal interactions among care receiver and caregiver, Musu also took significant satisfaction from observing the joy that the various educational and support therapies can bring:

> The best thing about this job is just watching and enjoying seeing the people [care recipients]. This morning, when I came in, one of the teachers who is in the music class had the other teachers play drums, because usually it's one of their goals [client goals, either set by themselves or as part of their plan of care] to learn how to play musical instruments, that's recreational. This morning, the teachers decided to play the melody for them, they were dancing. We just watch the way they are dancing happily, you just feel so, so fulfilled that really, they are enjoying life the way you want them to enjoy it, not to feel like their disability is hindering them from getting the joyful moments.

Michaela highlighted a different aspect of care that was satisfying: "To me, this job is like watching a baby grow up. When you watch your baby grow up, you see their steps changing. From helpless babies to when they are able to do something, it's like that. Some of these people come and they are unable to do anything, and then with a little training, a little training, we finally see that. That's why they must be praised for every effort that they make because it encourages them to want to do more."

While the comparison to babies is problematic, the essence of Michaela' words speak to patients' growth and accomplishment and caregivers' sense of pride and fulfilment. The following three quotations from Musu and Nelson, respectively, powerfully sum up the transformational process:

> I like the interactions that I have with the persons. Yeah, I really do enjoy that. Sometimes some folks [care recipients], we sit down and talk, some folks just sit and you just talking to them 'cause they are nonverbal; they don't hear anything. They are just sitting there, but you can tell it's just gonna crack jokes with them and stuff like that and they like that. They like that human touch. I think just for me, just that human touch, I think it's really very special with anybody. Who you are, you need that human touch. I think they, if they have enough of that, you can always tell the differences.
>
> When [care recipient's name], when he died, I was no longer working with him directly. But when he died, I cried. I missed him. I cried. This job has a way with the people you work with. They'll be a part of you in ways you don't even know. We'll be sitting there, with my cousins, with people who work here, we'll be sitting and talking and those are the things we'll talk about. Yeah, we'll talk about the old man, and he was so funny, et cetera, about the different relationships. It's just one of those things. We have very different relationships. We grow from it. I actually love my job [laugh].

I know it sounds like a cliché, but [the job has] made me a better person. With patients that I have now, in this job, when you have somebody who can spit on you and do these things on you, you're calm and you're OK. Or when someone's cursing you and you say I understand if you're upset.

As seen from these comments, disability support professionals who worked with clients with intellectual and cognitive disabilities in institutional settings, or in home settings brokered within their ethnic health labor markets, took pride in the fact that they could improve their charges' quality of life. This helped them get in touch with their humanity and apply universal principles of serving humanity to their work. The fact that they worked within settings controlled by and surrounded with coethnics also helped shape their overall positive experiences. Hawa Sesay, a Sierra Leonean house manager, expressed this sentiment when she stated proudly that working at Worldwide felt like "working for my own." Carole also said that one of the positive aspects of working at Worldwide was working with people of similar background, which made her feel "like it is home." Many workers in disability support also believed they had, themselves, grown because of their work. Albert articulated this: "I love working with people with developmental disabilities and it has helped me so much. I saw people in a different perspective. I actually saw how diverse the world is in terms of people in their social lives. Regardless of the fact that the people I was dealing with had some type of disabilities, I critically was able to sit down and look at a human being as a whole that to a certain extent, human beings, we all do have disabilities."

Many researchers have addressed emotional labor in care work and the depth of feelings and affect that caregivers and receivers can experience in this field that involves close and intimate relations. Some scholars have investigated emotional labor as a positive force that provides employees with dignity and rewards in a field that can be devalued (Rakovski and Price Glynn 2012; Showers 2018; Stacey 2011); others have analysed the exploitative nature of emotional labor when employers marshal employees' feelings to extract more labor or to justify poor treatment and remuneration (Diamond 1992; Dodson and Zincavage 2007). Sociologists Mignon Duffy, Amy Armenia, and Clare Stacey offer a related concept of "relationality," "the sustained emotional connection that may or may not take place in the context of paid work and that does not necessarily result in negative outcomes for the person(s) engaged in the emotional exchange" (Duffy et al. 2015, 8). The concept of relationality moves beyond the discussion of emotional labor and exploitation in care work to stress the reciprocal relationships engendered in a field that involves close and sustained emotional exchanges between two people. These relationships and bonds that can form between caregiver and receiver are "at once meaningful, personally fulfilling and also make workers vulnerable to burnout, emotional fatigue, or wage exploitation" (Duffy et al. 2015, 9). Relationality offers analytical insight to understand how West

African care workers I spoke with were at first sceptical to enter the field and faced both repulsion at performing intimate care tasks and the intrinsic rewards and positive feelings that came through their interactions and close bonds with care recipients with special needs.

These feelings were so strong that a few disability support workers, like Albert, Musu, or Joy, mentioned earlier, opted to remain in disability support, citing nonpecuniary reasons. As Musu said: "So, to me, if I were to be given a job that says I'm going to pay you more, I want the money, but I really want a job where I can interact on a daily basis with the people that I work with because I enjoy that." Musu explained further that she used her experiences in disability support to teach her children positive values and important life lessons. One of her sons, age twenty-three when I met her, had worked several summers at Worldwide, and she noted with satisfaction: "He got so attached to these people we work for." She went on: "My eight-year-old is also growing up, you know. I bring him around because, to me, these people need people that can be an advocate. We're not scared of them, we understand. I believe that bringing my son around teaches him from a young age that they're like me and you. They have things that they want. They have concerns. They have things that they want to do, just like you and I have. They have their own rights that should be met."

When asked to reflect on her career in disability support through the years, Musu concluded: "I wouldn't trade it for anything. Makes me say, you know, well, I guess nobody knows [what will happen] tomorrow. So, I want to treat them with my kids and let my kids know what I do. I always bring them [her children] to work, to see what we did. So, I won't trade it. I won't trade anything, 'cause I see this job, this individual, it's not the money. It's the passion. You have to care for this individual. If you don't have care for them, I don't know if you're wrong for this field or something, you must go to nursing home [you might be a better fit working in a nursing home]."

Exploring the world of disability support as mediated and brokered through West African-owned businesses has shown that the specific contexts within which care occurs (working in settings owned by coethnics versus mainstream institutions) and the specific care needs of care recipients (working with the intellectual disabled as opposed to exclusively with vulnerable older adults or the physically infirm) shape immigrant care workers' experiences. We have seen that while the work was generally difficult, dirty, and demanding, care workers took a lot of pride and gained intrinsic rewards from working with this segment of the care population. Working in ethnically owned businesses and surrounded by fellow West Africans provided an environment where disability support professionals could thrive, find meaning and dignity, and gain upward professional mobility. The care workers in this chapter were able to reconcile the class ambivalence they initially experienced and assess their success through non-pecuniary rewards. In the next chapter, I turn my analytical lens toward the experiences of those West African immigrants who made their way into skilled nursing professions and worked in mainstream institutional health care settings. Working within mainstream health care institutions and caring for a different clientele, including white and middle-class patients, meant that West Africans encountered a completely different set of circumstances and constraints, which we will now explore.

5 · PATIENT-PROVIDER INTERACTIONS AND PROFESSIONAL IDENTITIES IN NURSING

Lara Bello, an attractive, middle-aged, Nigerian registered nurse, sat across from me on a picnic bench in a public park on a Sunday afternoon. Like other care workers I got to know, she wore her smile and pleasant disposition as a shield. Yet I could hear a tinge of sadness in her voice even as her smile remained in place when she said:

> I found out in the beginning, being a foreign-trained nurse, and with [an] accent too, you meet all kinds of challenges. Patients, some of them would discriminate against who takes care of them . . . You might have some patient, who will tell you, "I can't understand what you are saying," "can you speak English?," "Can you just go back to Africa?" And some would not even tell you, but by their attitude you know they don't want you to take care of them. But going through that and seeing how the system works, where even though you are a charge nurse, because of the color of your skin, or because of where you are from, you are not so much recognized. You would have another person who is way below you and your manager might be giving that person instruction for the unit, instead of giving it you.

Lara went on to explain how she decided to combat such discrimination: "So, based on that, I just said, I have to go back to school. So, I went back to school to do my BSN and from my BSN, I went back to do my master's. Now, I am a master's prepared nurse, which is not so common. So that has placed me in a position where I feel I can do anything. If you don't respect me for who I am, you respect my certificate."

Using the experiences of nurses like Lara. in this chapter, I address African immigrants who had entered U.S. institutional health care settings, such as hospitals and nursing homes. While the disability support professionals in the previous chapter worked in settings predominated by coethnics, cared for a predominantly African American clientele, and gained mostly in intrinsic rewards (job satisfaction, positive affect, emotional connection to their charges), the nurses profiled in this chapter worked in institutional settings with a diverse workforce and encountered a more racially diverse set of care recipients. These nurses had made professional inroads in health care and gained in a combination of intrinsic (job satisfaction) and extrinsic rewards (professional mobility, material success). They also encountered unique challenges due to their work in mainstream health care institutions. I expand on the rewards of professional health care in the next chapter. Here, I pay special attention to how race and ethnicity shaped African nurses' encounters with patients, patients' family members, and colleagues, and how these encounters, in turn, shaped how they crafted their professional identities at work. I explore the strategies nurses used to navigate and combat their stated experiences of racism and African-origin discrimination in sometimes hostile work environments. This discussion reiterates the central argument of this book: structural gendered and racialized demands allow for concentration of Africans in entry-level positions and in the less-regarded and undesirable positions in professional health care contexts. In this chapter, I look at racism and workplace discrimination faced by respondents upon entering the professional ranks of the health care industry. I argue that Black immigrant professionals' experiences with racism and African-origin discrimination inform our understanding of the racial climate in health care institutions, racist organizational structures in health care, and identity formation processes among Black immigrants in the United States.

RACE AND GENDER AT WORK IN HEALTH CARE

When the nurses I spoke to described race relations in their workplaces, they often recalled confronting negative racial stereotypes in the course of their duties. Unlike their counterparts in disability support, who worked mostly in ethnically owned businesses, nurses in institutional settings or those who had worked in home care were more likely to report experiencing racism. These nurses also recalled specific instances—interactions with a patient, patient's family member, or a colleague or supervisor—that were negative and racist. Most identified statements, behaviors, and actions that they perceived to be racist. They also used the term "racism," except for one woman who simply referred to "Black/white problems." There were some, however, who were reluctant to name racism or interpret negative interactions using the language of race. A few expressed uncertainties about the role of race in negative experiences, especially with respect to incidents that could be understood as racial microaggressions.

In some cases, nurses reported that patients refused to accept care from Black health care workers. Sade Abiola, a Nigerian nurse, contextualized this problem:

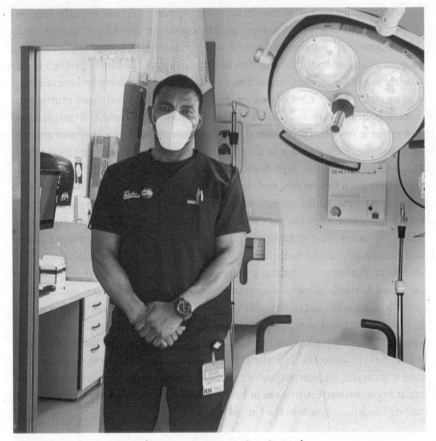

FIGURE 5.1. A nurse at work. (Photo courtesy Joseph Cole, RN.)

"Some of the patients are people you will sometimes get so connected to, they are like family to you. And some are mean; they don't even want you to touch them because you are Black." She recalled a particular incident:

> There was one particular case that stood out. The lady [patient] for some reason I don't know [paused], I went into the room and introduced myself to her and then a few minutes later, the charge nurse came to me and said that she will have to take that patient from me and give me another patient, and I said, what was the problem? I think she didn't really want to tell me what really happened because she didn't want to hurt my feelings. But apparently the family members said they didn't want me. So, they took the patient away from me.... They were Caucasians, so she took the patient away from me.

Sade's experience of racial tension with patients' family members was not unusual. While an explicit reason was never given for the patient's refusal of her service, Sade believed race was the issue, as she mentioned that the patient's family was "Caucasian." Mabel Mensah, an older nurse from Ghana, described negative interactions with disrespectful and demanding family members as a norm. She recalled that matters got so bad that "one day I told somebody: the slavery time has gone. We are working for you, and we respect you. . . . You need our services, we need your money, it's a two-way street. And we are doing the best we could for your mother, so I don't know what else you expect from us." The reference to slavery reflects Mabel's understanding that race plays a role in excessive labor demands placed on nurses. Nurses who interacted with patients' family members were more likely to narrate these negative instances. Henricia Gottfried, a Ghanaian nurse, said that families could be "very challenging in many ways." She described insults and some families being "downright rude."

Patients also questioned respondents' expertise. Maryam Barrie, a Sierra Leonean registered nurse, had recently lost a patient to cancer after caring for her in her home in her last months. She provided the patient intimate care, and she thought they had developed close relations and affective bonds. She was extremely hurt when her patient called in a white hospice nurse to care for her in her last days. Maryam felt that her patient had brought in "a white nurse to teach me my job." She also believed that her patient relied on and trusted the professional judgment and expertise of white nurses when it came to important matters and relied on Maryam only for the personal care and unpleasant tasks associated with that care. Maryam's interpretation that a white nurse was brought in because of their expertise and to provide instruction may very well be accurate—specialized hospice nurses have training designed for end-of-life care. It is notable, however, that Maryam interpreted her patient's actions as being motivated by race and racist notions that white nurses are more adept at the job than she is. She explained:

We used to have the hospice nurse who will come in and look at her . . . Because the hospice nurse is white, she will listen to her. Then I sat her down one day, and I said, listen, I have the same degree as she [the other nurse] does. Since you've been in this house [returned to her home after a hospital stay], have you ever been in the hospital because of an infection? She said no. I say because I take good care of you. I take care of you just as I would take care of my grandmother.

Here, Maryam was expressing a refrain that was common in the narratives of Black African nurses. These nurses felt that, as Black nurses, their authority, and expertise were constantly under threat and whiteness was automatically associated with professional competence, knowledge, and expertise.

Maryam's impression of her patient's disrespect reflects a culture in which Black nurses are routinely demeaned. In institutional settings, Black nurses and nurse managers often were mistaken for lower-level workers, while white aides were often assumed to be higher-level workers. Many nurse respondents reported being mistaken as nurses' aides by their white patients. A Sierra Leonean nurse manager reported an incident where a patient's relative walked past her seeking the nurse manager only to be referred back to her. As she said of the incident: "But they did not even bother to look at my badge, they just assume, they see this foreigner, she has an accent, how can she possibly succeed in this big hospital to be somebody up there."

These incidents suggest that patients and their families did not associate Blacks with professional status or positions of authority. These findings align with those of sociologist Adia Harvey Wingfield (2009), who unearthed a similar dynamic in which Black male nurses had been mistaken for janitors. Wingfield's findings, and my own, reflect a culture in health care institutions that does not recognize Black health care workers as suitable for professional grades in the health care hierarchy. The fact that the female participants here described being mistaken as nurses' aides and the males in Wingfield's study reported being mistaken as janitors highlight the intersection of gender and race in these instances. These gendered racist assumptions and stereotypes, or what eminent feminist sociologist Patricia Hill Collins (1991) has termed "controlling images," affect patients' and other actors' perceptions of and interactions with Black health care professionals.

Even administrators, who should recognize and acknowledge the qualifications of all workers under them, were not immune from these controlling images. Lara's story of a nurse manager who gave instructions for the unit to a lesser qualified nurse who was white, even though Lara was the charge nurse, was not unusual. Another nurse, Tosin Adesina, said that some of her department's administrators were "not fond of Black people." Many participants in this study described work environments and relations with fellow nurses on the floors of hospitals as "chilly." Mariama Bah, a Sierra Leonean registered nurse, believed that nurses in her unit, including native-born white and Black nurses and immigrant Asian nurses, refused to give her information relevant to a patient's care. She believed these nurses were setting her up to fail so she would be reprimanded by nurse managers. Rachel Owusu, a retired nurse from Ghana, recalled an incident that happened while she was still in nursing school. She had received a favorable decision from a review board after a white nursing instructor gave her a failing grade on a paper because she failed to type it. (This was before the use of computers became ubiquitous in higher education institutions). The overturn of the grade aligned with Rachel's feeling that racial prejudice was the reason behind the instructor's decision. These findings mirror studies of native-born Black nurses' experiences (Wingfield 2009, 2019; Ruchti 2012).

As Rachel's experience suggests, participants' experience of racial discrimination extended to their educational experiences, as well. Rose Asamoah, a Ghanaian nurse who had completed a bachelor's degree at a small, private, liberal arts institution before she went to nursing school at a prestigious institution in the Washington, DC, metro area, said that, while her undergraduate institution was primarily white, she felt othered at her nursing school where she was one of three people of color in her nursing class. She said that, being one of three people of color training to be a nurse, for the first time she had "actually felt being a minority." She went on: "But I guess having those experiences from undergrad, I sometimes forgot that I was colored, unless . . . some people used to make statements [paused] . . . you know at times when you sit down and think about it, it may cross your mind, could it be [because of race]? But I guess undergrad put me on a whole different level that I did not feel it as much."

Even though Rose felt that having previous experiences in a predominantly white undergraduate institution gave her professional advantage and the tools to deal comfortably with white people, her description suggests the presence of racial microaggressions that elicited sometimes visceral responses from participants.

Students at prestigious nursing schools and nurses at prestigious teaching and research hospitals are more likely to be white and to treat wealthy white patients (Dapremont 2013; Gillis 2010; Wingfield 2019; Phillips and Malone 2014). Unlike Rose, most of the nurses in this study had completed their education at community colleges or regional state universities and worked in nursing homes or the wards of regular hospitals that encountered more racial diversity among staff members and patients. Nurses like Rose felt the additional burden of being one of the few people of color in their classes or in their work environments. These nurses were more likely to report feeling a sense of isolation and experiences with racial microaggressions.

"MY ACCENT IS WHAT MAKES ME AN OBASANJO AND NOT A SMITH": ETHNICITY AND AFRICAN-ORIGIN DISCRIMINATION

In addition to race, ethnic identities were salient in African nurses' experiences in institutional work settings. The nurses believed that their ethnicity resulted in additional disadvantage in occupational settings and hierarchies. I conceptualize ethnicity here as a status that denoted their foreignness as immigrants to the United States and a specific identity as African-derived persons. Respondents from the five national groups often referenced their "foreign" or "immigrant" status and described themselves as "African" or "foreigner" instead of, or in addition to, their specific national origin status. This tendency likely reflects the impact of a U.S. culture that does not distinguish countries or ethnicities within Africa and that understands the vast and diverse continent as one single geographic mass. Patients, colleagues, and patients' family members with whom they interacted may very well be ignorant of or oblivious to the very complex national and ethnic differences among Africans.

The most common understanding of ethnicity among African nurses was that being African was disadvantageous in work settings due to stereotypes and pervasive negative views of the continent. Some nurses believed that native-born Americans associate Africa with economic and social decay, poverty, disease, ignorance, and other social ills. These negative views of Africa in the Western consciousness have been firmly established from Europeans' earliest encounters with Africans and are solidified in the present day through mass media portrayals and depictions (Ayisi and Brylla 2013; Pierre 2004; Morrow 1992).

More recent depictions of the continent as swarming with wars, political unrest, poverty, and disease (as evinced in the Western media coverage of health crises, such as the outbreak of the Ebola Virus disease in West Africa that lasted from 2014 to 2016) reflect similarly negative views of the continent.[1] These negative media portrayals of Africa and Africans in the Western imagination have shaped the way Africans are received in professional and social contexts (Beoku-Betts 2004; Beoku-Betts and Njambi 2005; Creese 2011, 2019). These entrenched portrayals of Africa as a backward continent, a lost continent, and the persistent white man's burden in the popular media were not lost on study participants. They believed these negative associations and stereotypes stigmatized them across various work settings and negatively influenced their interactions.

The women and men I interviewed recounted challenges to their sophistication, cultural capital, intelligence, and aptitude in performing their duties. Sharing phenotypic similarity with African Americans and other immigrants racialized as Black in the U.S. context, African immigrants described their distinct accents and speech patterns as the most identifiable features that marked them as Africans. Many had experienced negative reactions to their accents, which they felt hindered their care for patients and served as an obstacle to their professional mobility. A nurse who worked in an inner-city hospital, where most of the patients were African Americans, felt she had experienced discrimination that she did not think was "a race issue." It was "mostly when you open your mouth and speak, they know you are African so they are doubting whether this African can provide them with the care." This statement showed the complex intersection of race and ethnicity as, even in a Black-dominated space, Africans experienced negative reactions to their ethnicity as a distinct type of discrimination. The comment "Mostly when you open your mouth and speak, they know you are African, so they are doubting whether this African can provide them with care" is illustrative of the forms of contempt for Africans I am conceptualizing as African-origin discrimination.[2] Similarly, another nurse said, "My accent is what makes me an Obasanjo[3] and not a Smith," calling attention to the key role of accent in shaping respondents' unique experience as Africans.

Nurses who worked in predominantly white settings and prestigious institutions and specializations were very concerned that stigmatization of Africans would negatively affect their professional mobility. They believed they had to work harder than others to prove themselves. For example, Helen Johnson, a Sierra Leonean nurse working in an oncology unit of a large prestigious research hospital, said: "When I started [at the prestigious hospital] again it was another struggle between you being a foreigner, you having an accent, you being Black, you know, working at this hospital and working in this specialty . . . it was like a big thing. You know, I had a lot of obstacles when I first started, but I am a person, like I said, I do not give up and the more I see that you want to . . . bring me down, I fight a lot harder. It gives me more of a drive."

Even though Africans perceived that they were more disadvantaged compared to other Black racial groups, the belief that one had to work harder to combat racism and negative stereotyping is an experience shared with African American and Afro-Caribbean workers in health care and in U.S. society in general (Hine 1989; Wingfield 2019).

Mary Obasanjo, a Nigerian nurse, also experienced her accent as a reason patients doubted her expertise: "So, you meet a lot of patients, some of them look at you with your accent, and don't believe you can give them the care that they need. They doubt everything you do; your accent is a problem." She also noted: "On the contrary too, there were some that were appreciative of the care that they received."

Yvonne Doe, a Liberian nurse, reflected on the accent discrimination faced by African nurses. She had migrated to the United States with her parents at the age of five and, therefore, spoke without a discernible foreign accent. Due to her unaccented English, she often was mistaken as African American, and patients and their families would make candid and negative statements about the other African nurses in her presence. She explained that patients and their families would tell her that they had been unable to understand other nurses. She also expressed doubt that patients had really been unable to understand these nurses; as she noted, she had heard more recent immigrants who were "articulate" and "knew [their] stuff" and "said everything correctly," but "it just wasn't good enough because of that accent that was associated with it."

Arthurlina Stevens, who immigrated as an adult, had worked particularly hard to get rid of her accent. She said: "If you have an accent that's challenging, they think you don't know what you are saying or doing, so for me, I think I worked on my accent very quick, fast when I came in [to the United States]." Kate Yeboah, a Ghanaian nurse, explained how accent and race intersect in her experience: "There's a lot of racism and they are very prejudiced. I have lots of experiences to share with you, where people just see you and judge you. As soon as they see you, first of all you are Black. So, they think you are just a Black person from here, [the United States]. And then you start talking and it just puts them off."

These findings on accent discrimination mirror those of sociologist Gillian Creese. In a study of Black African immigrants in Canada, Creese (2011) found that in Vancouver, Canada, African English accents were marked as inferior and, along with other processes of racialization, proved to be obstacles to upward mobility for African immigrants. Across a range of job fields, Creese's middle-class and educated participants who were fluent in the English language prior to migration experienced accent-related prejudice, which she described as the "era-sure of linguistic capital." While many immigrants have accents marked as "for-eign," Creese's study participants perceived that their African accents marked them as distinct from and inferior to English, German, or French accents, for example. Likewise, the participants in this study believed their distinct accents and forms of spoken English were marked as inferior, even compared to Carib-bean English accents, in hospitals and other mainstream health care settings. Therefore, as Creese has argued, accents serve as a useful proxy to the racialized body where the African body is marked as particularly foreign, alien, and inferior (Creese, 2019).

Discrimination due to accents and the devaluation of Africans are associated with the erasure of human capital when premigration credentials are not recog-nized, as described in chapter 2, or as seen here, in the erasure of linguistic and cultural capital. In another study, Creese found that Black Canadians, regardless of citizenship or accent, were persistently met the query: "Where are you from?" As she described, this query is part of the process of racialization that mark Black bodies as foreign, strange, and out of place (Creese 2019). Sociologist Rhacel Parreñas notes that such queries work to make immigrants of color "perpetually foreign." In addition to reports of accent discrimination, some nurses I met also noted that repeated queries received from patients, such as "Where are you from?" or "When are you going back to your country?" made them feel perpetu-ally unwelcome.

Building on the work of Gillian Creese, I use African-origin discrimination to articulate the specific form of discrimination and disadvantage that is tied to people with recent migration histories from Africa. I posit that, along with skin color and other embodied/visible markers of identity (e.g., possessing so called "African features"), this form of discrimination is most immediately associated with "African accents" or African forms of spoken English. However, African-origin discrimination also could be triggered in contexts where Black bodies are read as foreign or unwelcome, as seen above, and especially when one's connec-tion to the African continent or recent African heritage becomes known.

Through African-origin discrimination, I attempt to name a phenomenon that has been identified by other scholars and to create unifying language to describe the disadvantage that Black African immigrants experience within vari-ous work contexts that cannot be explained only by their race and/or their status as immigrants: erasure of human, cultural, and linguistic capital; wage disadvan-tage relative to educational attainment; professional stagnation; employers' neg-ative perceptions of skill; negative reactions to accents; negative treatment by employers, co-workers, and others encountered within work setting; etc. (Beoku-Betts 2004; Beoku-Betts and Njambi 2005; Showers 2015a, 2015b; Tesfai 2019, 2021, 2020; Tesfai and Thomas 2020 Thomas 2014; Veit and Thijsen 2021). While African-origin discrimination is most pertinent to the experience of first-generation African immigrants, I leave open the possibility that this discrimination could be experienced by the second and subsequent immigrant generations without discernible "African accents" (Imoagene 2017; Creese 2019) if they have visual cues (e.g., style of dress, mannerisms) or other cues that are read as African-derived (e.g., African-sounding last names or in the cases where their African parentage or other heritage becomes known). In certain cases, African Americans or other Black people could be misrecognized as African, in which case they may be subject to African-origin discrimination in addition to anti-Back racism.

Structural Discrimination

As I have shown above, individual and interactional racism and African-origin discrimination exist within mainstream health care institutions. These forms of discrimination are situated on a continuum alongside more structural forms of disadvantage. Study participants felt that, in addition to facing racist treatment in interpersonal interactions, they face a racist system that limits their ability to advance their careers. They noted the concentration of African immigrants in nursing homes rather than in hospitals (which are better paid and considered more prestigious) and in specializations within hospitals that are more labor intensive, lesser paid, less pleasant, and considered less skilled. They also noted Africans are grossly underrepresented in managerial positions. These observations align with existing scholarship that has observed the presence of racialized hierarchies in the nursing industry (George 2005; Wingfield 2009, 2019; Raghuram and Kofman 2004; Yeates 2009).

Mariama, a nurse previously mentioned, who worked in a DC-area hospital, said that even though there are a lot of Africans who work on her floor, the charge nurses are all white. Likewise, she noticed a pattern where Black nurses were more likely to be assigned to the night shift as opposed to the preferable daytime shifts. Sociologist Adia Harvey Wingfield (2019) also documented this finding in her study of African American nurses. Mariama also felt that South Asian nurses would "work against" Black nurses "for the whites." Kate, a nurse mentioned previously, also felt that Asians had advantages over Black African nurses, noting that Filipina nurses get "more opportunities than Africans." These nurses' perception of a hierarchy that places Asian nurses above Blacks and below whites has been supported in other scholarship on nursing (Yeates 2009). A consensus that emerged among my interview participants was that, in a work environment stratified by gender, race, and ethnicity, Black, African, women nurses were at the bottom of all labor hierarchies. Highlighting the effect of ethnicity, participants felt that Caribbean Blacks had advantages over African

immigrants, and that African American women did, as well. Explaining the reason for her perception, that African Americans and other Black groups had
advantages over Africans, and, in fact, perpetuated African-origin discrimination, Harriet Williams, a Sierra Leonean nurse explained:

> Because they [African Americans], no matter what, they still think they are better
> than you. And I think that that has a whole lot to do with ignorance. That's my
> opinion, they still think that because you are from Africa, they are still better than
> you just because you are Black. And they believe, just because they have this
> American accent, in as much as you are more educated than they are, or have
> more degrees than they do, or more intelligent or more educated than they are,
> they still think that you know they are much better than you, just because they
> were born here, and you came from Africa.

Other nurses observed structural discrimination in nursing in terms of occupational specializations.[4] Being African was linked to professional stagnation and
subjugation in the least desirable and least regarded specialties, which I term the
"occupational ghettoes" of nursing. Participants noted that African immigrants
are overrepresented in less favorable specialties and faced obstacles to professional upward mobility. Sarah Josiah, a nurse practitioner from Liberia, gave her
assessment of race relations and racial hierarchies within nursing:

> If you are a Black woman working in the [Intensive Care Unit], they say wow,
> she's smart. And I don't think that should be the case. Everyone should be able to
> work there. Now, working in the nursing home when I worked as a CNA it was
> majority Africans. 'Cause most people don't want to do that work. Cause its
> quote unquote, it's a dirty job. So, it's the Africans, you know ... now it's the
> majority its Africans who work as CNAs. ... As a nurse in the telemetry unit, I
> found it was mostly African nurses. When I worked at the ICU, it was a different
> ball game. It was mostly Caucasians in the ICU.

Kate noted that she had known only a few Africans to hold positions of authority
in her workplace. Describing the case of one of the few African nurse managers
she knew, she said: "I used to work with this one lady, she was very competent. ...
She didn't last long ... I don't know, but she kept telling us the kind of problems she was having because she was a foreigner. ... You see [Africans] with
their master's still working on the floor. It's not like they don't qualify [for managerial positions]. But there is a lot of resistance, and sometimes they set them up
to fail. That's what I think, personally."

Kate's statement reiterates the sentiment held by many African nurses that
being Black and African not only exposed them to racial prejudice but also

limited their potential for advancement into the managerial and more prestigious ranks of the nursing field.

STRATEGIES TO COMBAT RACISM AND DISCRIMINATION IN THE WORKPLACE

To mitigate the negative effects of racism and African-origin discrimination they experienced, study participants enacted a few strategies. Respondents described trying to highlight their intelligence, caring personalities, hardworking personas, and professional orientations to work. They hoped that displaying these qualities to their patients and showing their sophisticated clinical skills would transform bigoted minds. For example, Yvonne said: "I think sometimes don't always look at the negative in things. If you say to yourself, I'm under advantaged. I'm Black, I'm African, I'm a woman, I'm this [pause] all your disadvantages, but you say I'm going to be the smartest, Black, African, youngest.... I was the youngest, Black, African. I was everything that was not the majority, and you know, and I just used it, like OK [pause] by the time I'm done taking care of you tonight and showing you my intelligence, clinical skills, etc., I bet you, you wouldn't think that again."

Many other interviewees referenced proving themselves or working hard to show their competence as the best approach to address racism. Kate explained:

Personally, what I have realized is, till you prove yourself, [patients] don't even want you. And it takes you to earn their trust. Because all my experience here [at a particular hospital], I realize that most people see you and even wish you were not their nurse just because you are foreign. But with time, at the end of the day, they come back to you, and they want you [pause] why? Because you have to prove to them that you know what you are doing. So, it makes very very . . . depressing sometimes. Feeling like you [are] not really welcome.

Thus, while Kate had learned how to work with patients whose initial impressions of her were based on bigotry, it took a toll on her emotionally. She continued: "I have a way I approach these patients, even as I'm saying they judge you right there when you get there. Even when you start nursing them, they realize that this is a different person. You have time for them, you listen to them, you taking care of their concerns, they know you have the skills, and then with time, they just start calming down and then then they change their attitude.... Most of them change."

Kate also worked hard to prove herself to bosses:

In terms of working with your bosses and stuff, sometimes they can also be very prejudiced. Especially when I was at the rehab hospital, the way they talk to you and stuff, they don't talk to the other, white nurses like that. So, I have the strong feeling that it's just because they prejudiced, they don't like you and they make life difficult for you. But even as I always say, I've had bosses like that and at the end of the day they have been my friends. Because I prove to them that I know what I'm doing. So, it takes that extra effort, although they judge you, to take that thing off their minds. But it can be really frustrating.

While Kate's narrative describes a happy ending in the form of a positive relationship with bosses who were initially racist, her words also reveal that Black and African immigrant nurses must perform an additional form of emotional labor to maintain a pleasant disposition and portray an aura of good grace that white and maybe other nurses of color need not perform.

Helen addressed similar themes when she said:

You find out that being a foreigner, being an African, having an accent... being Black, you have to work twice as hard as the white man for you to have that same position as the white man. You and the white man could have the same degree but he can go and just present his résumé/certificate or CV or whatever, and he can get the job, or even if you both have the same job, you always have to work twice as hard to prove yourself that you can do the job, and you probably, most likely ninety percent of the time, more intelligent or more educated than that other person.

When Helen uses "man" above, she is referring to universal humankind as translated from local Sierra Leonean language and not a gender identifier. "Working twice as hard" meant, for Helen, taking on additional tasks beyond what was required, or taking extra time in her duties to avoid making mistakes that would confirm stereotypes that she was incompetent or unqualified.

The nurses who worked in nursing homes used the term "working extra" to convey similar orientations, and to combat stereotypes of Black Africans as incompetent, unqualified, etc. The notion of "working extra" bears useful analytical weight to allow us to understand the additional labor costs and burdens that accrue to Black workers in health care and other professional settings. "Working extra" in these cases not only involves taking on additional work but also potentially subjects the worker to additional stress and emotional costs. These findings also align with those of Adia Harvey Wingfield (2019), who noted that African American health care professionals feel obligated to prove themselves more or work harder than white counterparts for the same rewards.

Additionally, within the context of care work, the idea of "working extra" bears interesting similarity to findings outlined by sociologist Clare Stacey (2011) in her study of home care workers. In that study of low-wage care workers, Stacey articulated what she termed "surplus care," where home care aides were asked to go above and beyond the call of duty to attend to their clients' need. "Surplus care" involved activities such as checking in on their clients outside of their paid hours, staying later than their allotted time slots to make dinner for a client, or taking on extra cleaning tasks beyond those specified by the terms of their contracts. Some aspects of "surplus care" also involved low-wage workers accruing financial burdens, such as paying for impoverished client's prescriptions out of their own pockets or lending money to their clients.

"Surplus care" allows us to understand the ways in which low-wage care workers, often with concomitant low occupational prestige, bear additional physical, emotional, and financial costs in the course of their work. It also adds an additional layer to the forms of exploitation that low-wage home care workers face that go beyond just low remuneration. While Stacey limited her analysis to workers at the base of the nursing hierarchy, the experiences of the nurses I have chronicled in this chapter show that while suffering from racial and ethnic disadvantage, Black, African nurses also were called upon to go beyond the call of duty in service of their patients. Here it is worth noting that, while the workers in this case were not explicitly asked to do extra work, they did so of their own volition to make their work environments and circumstances more bearable. "Working extra" shows that Black African immigrants in nursing, a high-status occupation in the health care hierarchy, suffered additional penalties, which may include performing additional tasks outside the purview of their contracted duties.

Beyond doing extra work on the job, interviewees described obtaining advanced degrees and specialized credentials to achieve upward professional mobility. While seeking additional credentials is commonplace in the nursing profession, in addition to advancing their careers, African nurses also viewed gaining more education as a strategy to combat racism and gain respect. When discussing their futures, many of the nurses, including a nurse who was approaching retirement age, said they meant "to go back to school." Lara, for example, described getting a succession of credentials to get respect. Reflecting her rationale, and referencing her absent colleagues, she said rather icily, "If you don't respect me for who I am, you respect my certificate." Similarly, Yenoh Sesay, a nurse participant from Sierra Leone, explained why she fought strenuously to get out of nursing assistant work where many other Sierra Leoneans were concentrated:

> For you to be taken seriously in life, you have to move on in life. I mean, you would see the difference the way they treat you when you are a CNA, and then, when you become an LPN. Even that big step, just that step that you've taken, the respect that you get from your bosses, is completely different from when you were a nursing assistant. Nursing assistant they treat you like you are an idiot, like you are a fool, that you are a low-class. . . . But when you improve yourself, one step, the treatment becomes completely different. Now they respect you, now they start taking you as somebody serious.

Arthurlina, a Sierra Leonean nurse manager previously introduced, explained how her education made a difference in how she was received: "I found it difficult when people didn't know my educational background. It's only when I whip out the educational card and give it to them, and they see the RN/BSN/MSN then they sort of look at you different.... So that's some of the challenges I've had, but when they realize my educational background, okay, you can see the ninety-degree turn [in their attitude]." Here, Arthurlina implies that she uses her educational credentials to combat patients' doubt about her expertise and competence. Sarah, the Liberian nurse practitioner previously mentioned, also stated: "So, as an African woman, as a NP right now, nobody discriminate [against] me. You know, I can go to any office, if I want to, and apply for a job. When I walk in as a NP, I get the respect. 'Oh, my goodness this is a smart woman, you know, she knows what's going on.' All my patients, I have white patients, I have Black patients, I have Asian patients, nobody will say 'I don't want you because you are Black.' They happy to receive care."

As these statements show, interviewees believed they could use educational credentials to buy insurance against racism and discrimination. A few who had arrived at the pinnacle of success in their nursing careers, such as the nurse practitioner and nursing home manager discussed above, believed this strategy was successful in combating racist prejudice and discrimination. However, the lived experiences of many more nurses I encountered showed the prevalence and persistence of interpersonal racial discrimination and structural racism in institutional settings.

Professional Distancing

In response to concentrations of Africans in the occupational ghettoes of nursing, and to be upwardly mobile in the profession, a subset of research participants engaged in a strategy I call "professional distancing." These nurses physically and discursively distanced themselves from coethnics in the profession, from work settings with large concentrations of other West Africans, and from "lesser-skilled" occupations in the health care industry such as certified nursing assistance.

In conceptualizing "professional distancing," I draw from sociologist Michèle Lamont and her discussion of the concept of "boundary work." This refers to the process by which certain groups assert their moral worth by drawing symbolic boundaries that define themselves as distinct from groups they do not belong to, based on racialized and gendered tropes that link work and dignity with moral characteristics. Among the West African immigrant nurses I interviewed, in response to the material and concrete realities they encountered in U.S. health care institutions and to the symbolism around nursing derived from their home countries, boundary work consisted of constructing physical and discursive boundaries between themselves and their coethnics at work.

There were a few reasons for engaging in professional distancing as a form of boundary work. One reason was due to premigration constructions of nursing in the home countries of Sierra Leone, Nigeria, and Ghana, in particular, as a vocation for women largely from poor backgrounds and with few other prospects. Nursing, in some cases, was viewed as unacceptable for women from "good families." Many of the Nigerian, Sierra Leonean, and Ghanaian nurses I met mentioned that nursing would simply not have entered their minds had they remained in their home countries. A U.S.-trained nurse originally from Nigeria confirmed these premigration orientations to nursing when she said: "Nursing in those days, used to be for those whose parents cannot pay for university education. That was how nursing in Nigeria . . . this is the mentality that we have. So, it wasn't like something I ever thought about doing."

Given this premigration background, nurses who had trained in their home countries, even when it was not profitable or prestigious to do so, characterized themselves as the "real nurses" and discursively separated themselves from their coethnics who had entered nursing in the United States. These nurses crafted their identities as "real nurses" for whom nursing was a "calling" in contrast to others trained in the United States, whom they cast as cold-hearted and calculating "opportunists" in nursing "only for the money" (Showers 2015b). Arthurlina reflected the views of those nurses who had trained in their home countries and the suspicion with which they viewed their U.S.-trained counterparts when she said:

And again, I'm not going to be biased, but for most of the folks who are entering nursing when they come to America, these are folks who, I look at them as opportunists for nursing, because you know, it's very difficult to get a job here [in the United States]. But I know friends who went to FBC [Fourah Bay College—a prestigious Sierra Leonean university], while I went to nursing school, and back in those days people looked down on you when you did nursing, especially in Freetown. They thought nursing was for the [high school] dropouts, so they all went up to FBC, of course, like I said from the onset, that was my calling. My other sisters all went to FBC, but I decided to go to nursing school. But when we come here, and I see them, doing nursing, I tend to think, why are you doing it? why the change? why didn't you start out with it from the get-go? Because of the financial benefits, as compared to back home and that's why I think a lot of people get into nursing when they come to America.

The loaded debate and charged accusations captured in Arthurlina's words, and the intensity of feeling between the "for love" versus "for money" camp in this research, reflect a more general debate in the theorizing and framing of care—a framing that often pits affect/emotion versus materiality in stark opposition to one another. I return to this debate in the next chapter.

In addition to these premigration orientations and divides, which were reflected mostly in the discourses of "real nurse" versus "opportunist," many nurses who engaged in professional distancing actively separated themselves from coethnics and/or areas in nursing where there were many other Africans. Helen employed professional distancing. She admitted that, in seeking work in the oncology unit of a nationally ranked teaching and research hospital, she was specifically seeking to avoid an environment that employs a lot of Sierra Leoneans. She saw the hospital that was "predominantly white" in terms of both staff and patient composition as a superior place for professional development, better than an institution or specialization employing more people of color. To get ahead in her profession, to "earn the highest income" she could, and to achieve utmost professional satisfaction, she said she had to "get away" from African immigrant colleagues to "get where I needed to go." By "getting away" from other Sierra Leoneans and seeking entry into an institution and specialization that was more prestigious and higher paid, Helen was seeking a strategy of advancement and upward professional mobility.

Harriet, another Sierra Leonean nurse, expressed similar sentiments. She described herself as having strong bonds in the Sierra Leonean community. She attended a Sierra Leonean church and was a frequent guest and patron at many community events. But at work, she said, "I decided to stay away from Sierra Leoneans." She had chosen to specialize in emergency nursing, a more prestigious specialty and one where she had only one Sierra Leonean colleague. A few other nurses, such as Rose, a registered nurse from Ghana previously mentioned, also engaged in professional distancing by enrolling in nursing degree programs at highly ranked and prestigious universities where few other Africans and, indeed, people of color attended. Others refused to start their careers as certified nursing assistants, which was, for most of the respondents in this study, their entry into the nursing profession.

While the nurses who engaged in professional distancing reported general professional satisfaction and more opportunity (better pay, higher occupational prestige) in prestigious, white-dominated workplaces, gaining entrée into these settings did not completely free them from the negative effects of race and ethnicity, as Helen experienced. She candidly explained that her immigrant status, her accent, and her race had been disadvantages when she first started at the oncology unit of a prestigious research hospital, and even after working in the field for many years, she felt she always had to work to prove herself. Further, as there were few other nurses of color in the workspaces she inhabited, she felt socially isolated. However, she framed these disadvantages as a motivator that made her "fight a lot harder" to get ahead.

RACE, ETHNICITY, AND BLACK IMMIGRANT INCORPORATION IN THE UNITED STATES

The racial experiences and identities unearthed in this chapter hold significance for our understanding of the integration of Black immigrants in the United

States. Professional distancing relates to the social distancing that scholars have found among first-generation Black immigrants who distanced themselves from African Americans to lessen the impact of racism (Arthur 2000; Foner 1987; Habecker 2012; Jackson 2010; Johnson 2008; Waters 1990, 2001; Vickerman 1999). These immigrants stressed their ethnic particularity and immigrant identities and culture to navigate U.S. racial formations and anti-Black racism. A line of scholarship has argued that employer preference for Black immigrants may be one reason for this strategy.[5] This distancing behavior and the question of whether ethnicity shields first-generation Black immigrants from some forms of racial discrimination have been widely debated in recent scholarship.[6]

I have shown that, rather than experiencing their ethnicity as an advantage, some African immigrants who suffered from severe disadvantages in institutional health care settings engaged in active distancing from coethnics and downplaying their ethnicity at work. Instead of experiencing preferential treatment from white supervisors, these immigrants experienced interactional racism and structural racism in mainstream health care settings. They also perceived that they were subject to negative stereotypes and discrimination by whites, other immigrants of color, and native-born African Americans. Thus, unlike some scholarship that has universalized the Black immigrant experience, this chapter points to heterogeneity among Black immigrants. I have argued that the social construction of the regions and nations from which Black immigrants derive, including popularized media images, stereotypes, and meanings associated with regional origin, shape their reception at work. Professional contexts, including the particularities of specific occupations; the social organization of workplaces, including the racial, ethnic, and national composition of the workforce; and the histories and contexts of local geographies also shape integration. For instance, urban policy scholar Faranak Miraftab (2016) explored the racial hierarches in Beardstown, Illinois—a small town in the rural heartland of America dominated by a Cargill industry-owned meat-packing plant. She focused on the experiences of Latinx immigrants primarily from Mexico and Central America, Black West Africans primarily from Togo, and a sample of African American internal migrants from Detroit. In this primarily blue-collar setting, crippled with the social effects and economic displacements of deindustrialization, highly educated French-speaking West Africans from premigration middle-class backgrounds with legal immigration status ranked higher in whites' estimation than African Americans and Latinos, who were racialized as "illegal immigrants." African Americans ranked at the bottom of the racialized social hierarchy in that context. Miraftab concluded: "While Africa may be stigmatized as the 'dark continent,' the reputation of Detroit—as a rust belt city of 'crime and thugs' does not advance the position of African American Detroiters in Beardstown" (Miraftab 2016, 74). In hospitals and nursing homes in metropolitan Washington, DC, and in the nursing field, which contains intimate exchanges and close physical contact, what I think of as "tactile proximity," among different racial/ethnic groups, Black "foreigners" from Africa with "strange" accents ranked at the bottom of professional hierarchies.

I also have shown that, through professional distancing, some West African nurses, like Helen, equated whiteness with success in the world of work and explored strategies to enter white-dominated fields. However, I did not find that this distancing behavior extended beyond work settings, and, in fact, several of the nurses were actively involved in their immigrant and coethnic communities. These findings that Black immigrants seek admission into the socioeconomic mainstream do not, however, negate the significance of race or racial inequality in U.S. society. As I have shown, African nurses clearly understood racial hierarchies and racial discrimination as problems that they faced in professional health care contexts. This chapter has, therefore, pointed to a paradox for Black African immigrants who are racialized as Blacks in the U.S. racial context and experience racial discrimination but also employ professional distancing and other strategies of assimilating into whiteness (seeking entry to white-dominated spaces and institutions) to gain upward mobility. These strategies of assimilating into white spaces yield limited results, as they still suffer from the effects of racism and African-origin discrimination at the interpersonal level.[7] In the next chapter, I examine the issue of success and upward mobility among Black African immigrants within the context of work in health care occupations. How can we assess and measure success of this immigrant group, and what does this all mean for U.S. society broadly speaking and health occupations in particular?

6 · NURSING A PATHWAY TO THE AMERICAN DREAM

When someone goes to school, you're looking at the job. You're looking at what your future is going to be looking like. But then in Africa, it was kind of like bleak. But when I came to the United States, I started feeling a sense of my future, what it's going to look like, whether or not I'm going to be able to sustain myself and get a family and call myself a dad or something. All of those things have to come when you are settled down, and I saw that kind of settlement when I came to the United States.

—Sheikh, administrator at Worldwide

What I want to do after I finish my PhD, because I would love to do it in macroeconomics and public health, I would go back to Sierra Leone as a politician. That's what I want. To go back to Sierra Leone, as a politician, to influence the mental health field. Africa is not doing well in that area. We are neglectful of people's lives. I was astonished to see that America has a system where you're helping people with challenges. They house them, they feed them, they clothe them, they care for them. Africa doesn't have that. It is taboo to have somebody in your family who has an intellectual disability.

—Albert, QIDP at Worldwide

I'll be happy if my eldest daughter who is now in school [becomes a nurse]. She was trying to do LPN. I'm going to encourage her to do more. I really would like for [my other children] to do something more in assisting people. Whatever it is, be it group homes, or be it healthcare business like home healthcare, I just want them to know that giving a helping hand is the best they can do in this world. You'll be blessed with that.

—Anwar, administrator at Heath Care Agency

The immigrant "success story" often is framed around the trope of the American dream.[1] In this framing, immigrant success is measured by professional attainment, education, income and wealth accumulation, home ownership, and entrepreneurship. These financial measures are sometimes assessed alongside social and political metrics like language acquisition, assimilation into mainstream social institutions, naturalization rates, intermarriage rates, and so on. Other times, success is measured in the achievements of the immigrant second generation. For example, did they surpass the achievements of their parents in earnings, educational attainment, and mobility into the professional class and out of the ethnic niches of employment occupied by their immigrant parents? And did they successfully integrate into American nationhood? (Alba and Nee 2003; Dhingra 2012; Imoagene 2017; Louie 2012; Portes and Zhou 1993; Portes and Rumbaut 2014; Zhou and Bankston 1998).

How do we measure the success of African immigrants in health professions and in U.S. society writ large? And what does success mean for their children? Earlier chapters have shown workers' paths of mobility out of the "dirty work" of care to professional ones, as nurses in hospitals and nursing homes, and jobs with increased authority and responsibility in ethnic-owned businesses. Some even had achieved moderate success as entrepreneurs in home care and disability support, albeit in a lower-tiered and marginalized market. Yet, the previous chapter described the difficulties some nurses faced in mainstream health care settings (racism, African-origin discrimination, hostile work environments). To make sense of these contradictory trends of initial downward social mobility after migration, professional mobility, and opportunity in some segments of the health labor market and discrimination in others, I turn to analytic tools in the two major bodies of literature that I have engaged in this book: the sociological literature on U.S. immigration and the interdisciplinary literature on paid care work.

Researchers who study paid care work also have long debated the merit and worth of these jobs. "How much is care worth?" is a difficult question, given it encompasses the labor of family members who might be compensated to care for loved ones to paraprofessional nursing assistants in institutional settings, paid childcare workers, teachers, skilled nurses, and so on. Many studies of care work tend to highlight low compensation; job insecurity; lack of or inadequate benefits such as sick leave, health insurance, workers compensation, and retirement plans; little professional mobility; overwork and burnout; and exposure to workplace injury, sexual harassment, and racism as central characteristics, especially for lower-wage workers in home care and institutional elder care (Boris and Klein 2012; Covington-Ward 2017; Coe 2019; Diamond 1992; Duffy 2005, 2007, Foner 1994; Osterman 2017; Rakovski and Price Glynn 2010; Stacey 2005, 2011; Schweid 2021). Accounts of nursing, better paid and further up the professional ladder, also show problems with workplace injury and burnout, as well as the persistence of racism, xenophobia, sexism, sexual harassment, and abuse by co-workers, patients, and patients' families (Wingfield 2009, 2019; Hine 1989; Ruc-thi 2012; Showers 2015a).

The challenges and constraints of care occupations are clear, but so are the benefits and the rewards. Drawing from the experiences of home care workers, sociologist Clare Stacey (2005), for instance, understood intrinsic rewards—job satisfaction and fulfillment gained from and through the altruistic caring for others—as a mechanism through which workers import dignity to marginalized work. These rewards allow workers to stay on the job, at least in the short term, despite its constraints. At the same time, while gaining much in terms of intrinsic satisfaction, these workers are vulnerable to frustration (Stacey 2005, 2011). Other studies have documented the use of religious tropes of "sainthood" that workers use to frame their work as caring, altruistic, and motivated by love even as they face humiliation, shame, degradation, and poor material rewards (Coe 2019; Solari 2006; Zelizer 2005). Anthropologist Cati Coe articulated the concept of "divine reciprocity" among some of the African immigrant home care workers she studied, who turned to otherworldly and religious framings of their expectation of rewards to cope with the challenges of their jobs. Many studies similarly report descriptions of care work as "a calling" and articulations of doing "God's work" (Solari 2006; Stacey 2011) as ways to make difficult jobs bearable and rewarding. Focusing on more worldly concerns, a study of frontline health workers, for instance, reported that these workers have high job satisfaction but are likely to leave their jobs (Morgan, Dill, and Kalleberg 2013). The empirical emphasis on mostly low-wage, low-prestige care jobs has led to positioning intrinsic and extrinsic rewards as dichotomous and conflicting, with intrinsic rewards serving as compensation for the lack of extrinsic rewards. Yet, as the previous chapters have shown, for many Black African immigrants to the United States, care jobs provided extrinsic rewards. These include a point of entry into the labor market, a livelihood, and, for many, the opportunity to send remittances home. Compared to other entry-level immigrant employment niches, such as the food industry or agriculture, many respondents found care jobs to be better paid with more autonomy and flexibility.

Wages earned from direct care work and nursing were salient as extrinsic rewards for West African care workers. Cati Coe's research on African immigrants also emphasized the importance of wages, even the relatively low wages earned by home care workers. Those wages, while low for the United States, still presented as an extrinsic reward when compared to opportunities in the home country. A home care worker Coe interviewed said of fellow home care workers: "They don't look at" a job's hardships. "They look at the money. They have pressure back home, from children's school fees, or [a sudden need arises such as] someone dies [and they have to pay the funeral expenses for a relative]" (Coe 2019, 220–221). Many of my interviewees, similarly, mentioned money when I asked them questions about the positives of the job. Indeed, "Nurses make money" was a common refrain. As Albert, the Sierra Leonean former university lecturer, stated, becoming a disability support professional allowed him to put "bread and butter on the table."

The drive "to make money" might seem to contradict the claim that workers in this area are altruistic or saints, as well as the reality of low wages in many segments of care work. I unpack this paradox in two ways. First, many of the care workers I met, (both lower wage paraprofessional DSPs and the highest paid professional nurses), embarked on income augmenting strategies to increase hourly pay rates. Second, beyond survival and funding remittances, many used their wages to increase their human capital, paying for further schooling or credentials that helped launch their careers in professional segments.

In terms of income augmenting strategies, many care workers I encountered worked at least two jobs with different employers. Nurses, for instance, worked daytime hours at a hospital and overnight shifts as a home care nurse or weekend shifts at a different hospital. While nurses make decent wages even by U.S. standards,[2] many embarked on these income augmenting strategies to fund the lifestyles they had adopted after successfully training as nurses. I expand on these material lifestyles later in the chapter. Such strategies take a toll, as I came to realize when I phoned Kezia, a licensed practical nurse from Liberia, on a Sunday evening. She told me she had been working continuously since I had seen her that Friday afternoon. It was not uncommon for interviewees to report in phone conversations that they had completed double or consecutive work shifts. Many, especially those at the lower end of the spectrum, worked sixty- to eighty-hour weeks to extend low hourly wages.[3] DSPs and those who had worked as home care workers opted for live-in employment, another strategy to maximize funds, as it saves on housing costs.

Cati Coe also found evidence of overwork among her interlocutors. She described a research participant who said that live-in work can encourage never taking time off work, and (perhaps with some hyperbole), "some people die" because they never take a break (Coe 2019, 221). Some of the administrators of recruitment agencies I met that hired mostly African immigrants told me that their main reason for dissatisfaction with their staff was that they were working too many hours with other employers and this impaired work performance. A few nurses of the immigrant 1.5 generation also described overwork as a problem with first-generation immigrants. They described these work practices as contributing to nurse burnout and believed they negatively impacted their clinical practice. For their part, care workers reported physical and emotional exhaustion, burnout, chronic stress, and related health outcomes such as high blood pressure and injury, especially back injuries, as some of the most difficult aspects of their work.

The strategies devised to increase hourly pay rates provide some context for understanding how remuneration or financial rewards became significant for

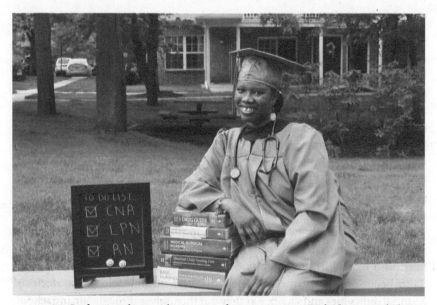

FIGURE 6.1. Graduation photo with associates degree in nursing. Such photos symbolize the prestige that nursing degrees signaled to members of the West African immigrant community. (Photo courtesy Charann Caulker, RN.)

West African immigrants. Money held several symbolic and practical meanings for the participants in this research. For the nurses, especially, money earned from direct care work translated into the ability to pay for their credentials and licenses in nursing. "To pay for school," as many put it. In moving out of direct care work to more advanced licensures in health care, care workers outlined a step-level process; that is, moving from one gradation in health care to the next, saving money to help pay the cost for education and licensing for the next stage. Indeed, many of the nurses I interviewed had taken this route, starting as CNAs or HHAs and enrolling in part-time classes at local community or private two-year colleges, to take additional classes. Figure 6.1, a photograph taken at a nurse's graduation with an RN qualification from a local community college, illustrates this stepwise path of mobility in health care work.

A common strategy used to balance work and education was to work overnight shifts, which allowed nurse trainees to take daytime classes and then care for a patient while simultaneously studying and doing homework during the night. Sade, a Nigerian nurse who was the director of nursing of a home health agency, recalled deploying this strategy while working as a home health aide and studying to be a nurse: "So, while I'm with the client in the house, she may be sleeping, I could take my book and read."

Tuition costs were a huge factor in the choice of educational institutions. Some nurses explicitly stated that they deliberately chose cost-effective options, such as starting out at community colleges or enrolling in less-expensive four-year colleges. Harriet, a Sierra Leonean-trained nurse who retrained in the United States, recalled how she sacrificed and saved her wages earned as a certified nursing assistant shortly after arriving in the United States: "I have to do whatever it takes [to become a licensed nurse in the United States]. I actually took my NCLEX [nurse licensing exam] in New York. So, I struggled. It got to the point where I was saving every dime that I had. Sometimes I just drank milk for the whole day, just so that I would be able to go to review school. I went to the review school for a whole week, I went to New York, stayed in New York for a couple of days, and then took my NCLEX."

Earning and putting away money to pay for the next licensure was common, and as Harriet illustrated, the path from direct care work to registered nurse was filled with difficulties and a lot of sacrifice. Other nurses, such as Yenoh from Sierra Leone, who had earned a master's degree in nursing, told similar stories of financial difficulties and sacrifice as they put themselves through nursing school. Yenoh said:

> I went to school without even having books, textbooks. I remember, my husband and I, I met my current husband at school. So, we had like four [younger classmates] in the program. So, I mean most of the time I will take their textbook, make copies of the chapters, and then that's how I would get my books. . . . At that time things were hard. I didn't have any textbooks. I had my daughter. I had to sponsor, I mean, pay the lady taking care of her, because I couldn't take care of her. I didn't have a car, I didn't have anything, so I had to leave her with an aunt, that I used to pay like $300 a month, plus my rent, plus my responsibility back home. So sometimes I would end up with like $20 for the next two weeks.

Like Yenoh, many other nurses spoke about the difficulties of financing their educations. Most, like Harriet and Yenoh, used monies obtained from direct care jobs to start. Nurse X,[4] an LPN at Worldwide, described that she started her associate's degree one class at a time until a windfall from an annual tax refund allowed her to pay for a year's full-time tuition at once. A few, largely those who went to four-year institutions, took out student loans to finance their education. Describing this funding strategy and the struggle to repay those loans, Rose, a registered nurse, who had earned a BSN at a prestigious university, said, "The bill is sitting there waiting." In other words, like millions of Americans, these nurses seemed to be saddled with student loan debt.

Starting from CNA or other areas of direct care work and progressing up the nursing ranks also was captured within the orbit of social media. Upon completing their degrees, West African nurses posted professional-looking and staged

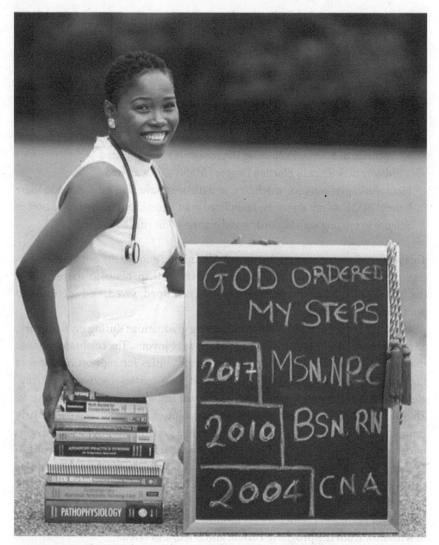

FIGURE 6.2. Graduation photo with master of science in nursing. Like many nurses in the study, Andrea Rex-Campbell started out as a CNA, then pursued further credentials in a stepwise progression. (Courtesy Andrea Rex-Campbell, MSN, FNP-C. Photographer: Alhaji S. Kargbo.)

graduation photos and wrote touching tributes to those who had supported them. They posed with cap and gown, or in fashionable outfits, with graduation cords around their necks and nursing textbooks in hand or within the frame. They sometimes stood proudly next to a chalkboard, with the steps along the nursing hierarchy listed in a stepwise order, and accompanying boxes checked off in large and colorful checkmarks (see Figures 6.1 and 6.2).

The following words of a Facebook post by a Sierra Leonean nurse celebrating her graduation with a master's degree capture the sense of accomplishment, but also the stepwise professional journey beautifully:

> Life is a process, not an event. Everyone's path will be different, and this is my path:
>   Certified Nursing Assistant (CNA)—Completed
>   Licensed Practical Nurse (LPN)—Completed
>   Associate Degree in Nursing/Registered Nurse (ADN/RN)—Completed
>   Bachelor of Science in Nursing Degree (BSN)—Completed
>   Master of Science in Nursing Degree (MSN)—Just arrived.
> Hard work, perseverance, discipline, and blessing have allowed me to add these letters "MSN" to my signature, completed grad school, and received a Master of Science in nursing with leadership and management concentration.

This joyful tribute to success, hard work, discipline, good luck, and divine blessings captures the sentiments of many research participants who started out at the bottom of the health care industry then scrimped, saved, and sacrificed to put themselves through school.

I attended three parties celebrating nursing graduations during my fieldwork, all for women. These graduation celebrations were joyous. The celebrants offered thanks to God, their families, and larger communities for supporting them as they pursued their goal. The speeches given at these parties discussed the struggles they faced in balancing work and childcare and also taking nursing classes. They described the coursework as challenging. One of the nurses was particularly candid about the failure she had experienced in a previous attempt to qualify as a nurse while caring for her newborn baby. I recorded this quote in my field notes: "When I went to the University of Maryland. . . . At the time [child's name] was six months. . . . I took care of my baby as best I could, trying not to fail. But talk about hopelessness. My very first semester, I failed pathophysiology and had to take it over again. . . . I went back six months later, and then I failed again and had to withdraw from the program. I cried, and cried, and cried."

She then talked about the difficulty she faced to gain admission to another program, having failed out of the first program. She credited her eventual success to God, the help she received from a kind nursing dean who gave her a second chance, her family, and support systems. In this and the other graduations, the success being celebrated was framed as a communal success in which everyone in that immigrant community should take pride.

It became clear through these graduations and other interactions among West African immigrants that those who had succeeded in moving from direct care work to professional nursing commanded a lot of respect and admiration in their immigrant communities. In addition to being hailed as professional successes, nurses had become an emblem of the American dream as measured in material terms—home ownership and conspicuous consumption of luxury items such as expensive cars, clothing, and, sometimes, enviable travel. Once when I met up with a registered nurse from Liberia at a local coffeeshop, I was impressed when she arrived in a sleek black Mercedes Benz. I visited the homes of many nurses as I conducted interviews, and I observed that many registered nurses, and the few nurse practitioners, owned impressive homes with soaring ceilings, expensive furniture and décor, and, for some, luxury cars parked in driveways.[5] The younger nurses mostly lived in shiny, newly built suburban subdivisions, while older registered nurses, mainly from Ghana and Nigeria, were more likely to live in more established neighborhoods.[6] Younger licensed practical nurses were more likely to live in modest townhomes[7] or apartment complexes. Sociologist Anna Guevarra also found an understanding of nursing as a pathway to the American dream among Filipina immigrant nurses. Filipina nurses in Texas and Arizona interviewed by Guevarra also espoused an Americanized view of success measured in part through the heightened power to consume material goods: homes, cars, and other possessions. These nurses also gained heightened social standing among their families in the homeland, who ascribed them new roles as "economic providers, gift givers, success stories in their families" (Guevarra 2010, 169).

That many West African nurses I interviewed, like the Filipina nurses studied by Guevarra, had been able to purchase and maintain sizeable homes, often in racially integrated suburban neighborhoods, is in stark contrast to the findings of anthropologist Cati Coe. The dream of home ownership eluded the African elder care workers she studied in suburban Maryland and northern New Jersey. Not only were they often unable to purchase homes, but when they did so, they struggled to maintain mortgage payments because of the precarious conditions and contingent nature of agency-brokered home care jobs. Coe writes: "Although home ownership may result in middle class status, home ownership among the African care workers I knew was often a source of wealth extraction" (Coe 2019, 2). Indeed, a key informant in her study lost her home to foreclosure.

The overarching picture painted by Coe was that African immigrant elder care workers were shut out of the American dream, in material terms and in emotional and affective terms. Barred from the material benefits of citizenship and "political belonging" in America, the care workers Coe interviewed devoted their energies and their incomes to home building projects in their home countries with cheaper housing markets (Ghana, in particular). Rather than reaping the rewards of decades of work, Coe writes, "ten to forty years after arriving in the United States, they felt disappointed by the American dream" (2019, 204). This was far from the experience of West African immigrant care workers I got to know. Not only had they bought into the American dream hook, line, and sinker, at least in the case of nurses, they appeared to have reaped some of its material benefits.

While evidence of financial rewards and success abound through my own observations of the material possessions of nurses and, as previously noted, through general statements made by other care workers, due to my in-group membership and the sensitivity of talking about finances, I did not ask direct questions about wages earned in dollars and cents. The nurses were more likely to stress the importance of wages to their professional mobility and as a reward of their hard work. Apart from Kate, a Ghanaian registered nurse, who told me she had earned $180,000 one year (by working in more than one job),[8] and Yvonne, a Liberian nurse supervisor for a local school district, who had two master's degrees, who told me she had negotiated a $130,000 salary, interview participants did not give me specific details about salaries earned or discuss their success in materialistic terms. The material signs of their success were, however, quite visible, as I have shown.

Those immigrants who had become nurses seemed to have "arrived," and their communities viewed them as living the American dream as measured in their possessions. How they afforded these lifestyles, however, is worth reiterating. They did so through working many hours at multiple jobs, and often working unfavorable weekend and night shifts, which allowed them to earn overtime rates (higher than the prevailing hourly wage rate). When one considers the costs of overwork to their physical, psychological, and emotional health, as well as their family life, one can conclude that success for West African immigrant nurses came at the price of reasonable rest, recreation, self-care, family life, and other quality of life measures.

I never visited the private homes of disability support workers, conducting those interviews at offices or the group homes they staffed, so it is not clear whether they had homes, fancy cars, and other material trappings of the American dream. Disability support professionals do earn lower incomes than registered nurses and nurse practitioners.[9] Many had migrated as adults and almost always had encountered downward social and occupational mobility after moving to the United States. They became DSPs after pivotal moments of great disruption in their personal and professional lives in the United States, and sometimes after trying out other low-wage and low-prestige service-oriented jobs. Unlike the nurses, some had not received any education in the United States. Most worked in businesses owned by coethnics (most at Worldwide), and they emphasized that they were climbing the promotion ladder at work. Rather than emphasizing wages, they viewed the opportunity for growth and upward professional mobility they had been able to achieve at Worldwide as a reward of their jobs.[10] They also appreciated that the management at Worldwide were willing to overlook their lack of U.S.-earned credentials.

Augustine, who had taught high school math and science in Sierra Leone, explained proudly that he had started from the "grassroots" to progressing to now being a supervisor in disability support. He described a process in which, after starting out as a hands-on caregiver who provided personal care and direct support at the day program and residential settings, he skillfully cultivated relationships with his co-workers and managers. By developing a spirit of cooperation and acquiescence, he slowly moved up the ranks to the point where he came to hold a supervisory position as a qualified intellectual disability professional. In his description of the climate at Worldwide, opportunities became available as his coethnics also climbed up the professional ladder.

As described in chapter 4, QIDPs and house managers at Worldwide went through powerful transformations and gained intrinsic rewards as they adjusted to their caregiving roles in disability support. While developing empathy and affection for those in their care and inner satisfaction in their jobs, disability support professionals who, like Augustine, had moved from direct support roles also experienced the status that came with their supervisory roles as an extrinsic reward of their jobs. Albert, a Sierra Leonean QIDP, who was conspicuous in his professional dress and demeanor, described with pride the advantages and responsibilities inherent in his move from being a direct care worker to case manager at the day program and then to QIDP in the residential homes:

At that point in time [as a case manager], a major advantage was that you have a number of people you're responsible for, and staffed under you, whom you supervise to ensure that the ISP [Individual Support Plans] have been implemented. And also, active treatment, in particular, was done as specified. And also, I was responsible to liaise, or to link, or coordinate service with different providers in terms of physicians' orders, consultant notes. And then you will benefit the people supported at that time. If you see [a care recipient] come [to the day program who doesn't] look very much. . . . well cared for, I will report that to DDS [Department of Disability services] or call the people in charge and talk to them. It is important to have nice shave or haircuts, and fingernails [should not be] dirty. I will always be responsible for reporting those things.

He described the enhanced responsibilities of a "Q" thus:

As a Q, it's more of an expansion of being a case manager. You have additional tasks attached to your functions. Now, all the work that we do in the day program, a Q does, does more. Like coordinating, you have staff under you. You have a house manager, and you coordinate with family members, the attorneys, guardians, service coordinators, Department of Health, Administrative office. So, that is an expansion. An expansion at the facility level, you coordinate, you liaise with the administrative office. You work with DDS. You work with service coordinators. And the attorneys, guardians, and you go to court if people you support are court admitted. You go to court to overview their well-being.

Albert loved the fact that he was no longer a direct care worker but was now in a position to be an advocate for the well-being of his clients. He took pride in his role in preventing neglect of care recipients and reporting potential incidents to the powers that be. Nurse managers and charge nurses expressed similar sentiments.

I have argued thus far that a significant number of West African immigrants who were produced, repackaged, and deployed as care workers after migrating to the United States also gained extrinsic rewards: upward mobility from direct care work, relative financial success, and increased responsibility and authority. Even though they experienced difficulties, as previous chapters have shown, they also gained in intrinsic rewards. For example, Lara, a Nigerian registered nurse we met in chapter 5, said: "I am not one of those [people], that will say, oh I entered nursing because I like caring for people and all that. No, it was not that, it was not in my—nursing was not in my agenda at all. I didn't want to do it initially, but today I'm glad I did. You know sometimes, we do things that you think people are forcing you to do or something like that, but you find out that this is actually where you should have been a long time, and I enjoy it. I can't even do anything else."

Lara had become a nurse because the field provided a livelihood and immigration status benefits in the UK before her migration to the United States. While she rather controversially stated that she did not enter nursing because she "loved caring for people and all that," she also said, "I didn't want to do it initially, but today I'm glad I did . . . I can't even do anything else." Lara's experience is like others in the literature on care work. Paula England, Nancy Folbre, and Carrie Leana (2012), for instance, reported similar discussions among research subjects; in one case, a grandparent who was forced to care for their grandchildren but eventually developed satisfaction or love of their caring role. Similarly, Yenoh said she had continued to do bedside nursing even though she had opportunities to be in a supervisory role because: "I really love it. . . . Because the idea of helping somebody, knowing that you have contributed in somebody's life, or you have helped somebody to die with dignity, really gives you the satisfaction." Many nurses described their job as "fulfilling." Many had grown to love their jobs more the longer they stayed on the job.

Even nurses who had viewed their paths into health care as temporary reported intrinsic rewards. Rose, a Ghanaian registered nurse, initially had wanted to be a doctor but had failed to get into medical school. She also sought admission into graduate programs in public health before settling on nursing. She said, however, that going into nursing was "the best decision I ever took." She reflected:

I feel like at the end of the day, I'm still at the point where I know that I am making a difference in someone's life. And that's always what I wanted to do. I mean, working with people and helping to make that change. I mean, I could have possibly done that in a different way, working in an office somewhere, but this is where it's like, you are there with the people, helping people out, and that is pretty much what I wanted to do when I was in [college] and when I wanted to go into medicine or public health. But then with nursing, this is more of patients and people who are sick, sick, sick.

Rose had no plans to seek a different career, and this was common. Almost all the nurses described plans to "go back to school" to gain further credentials in nursing. When I caught up with a few for follow-up interviews, or followed their progress on social media, I found that a few had, indeed, succeeded. For example, Rose would later become a nurse practitioner, and Temi, a Nigerian RN/MSN, would earn a doctorate in nursing practice a few years after our initial interview.

Theorizing the intersection of intrinsic and extrinsic rewards in care giving occupations, economist Nancy Folbre and sociologist Erik Olin Wright wrote, "love and money often combine and intersect sometimes though not always in complementary ways" (Folbre 2012, 2). West African immigrant professional care workers (nurses and disability support professionals) gained a combination of extrinsic and intrinsic rewards. For them, love and money did work in tandem. They also had come to develop what Folbre and Wright term "prosocial motivations" or the "concern for the well-being of others." However, contrary to Folbre and Wright's assumption, they had not always entered care giving roles because of "prosocial motivations that offer intrinsic rewards, such as the gratification of helping others or the genuine desire to make the care recipient better off" (Folbre 2012, 3). Rather, some developed the motivation "to help others" after being immersed in their jobs and having gained knowledge from many years working in U.S. health care settings and institutions. They expressed this knowledge in biomedical terms. For example, Arthurlina, a Sierra Leonean registered nurse and nursing home administrator, described diagnosing ailments after family members described symptoms over the phone. Nurses like Arthurlina felt they would be able to help their family members and their immigrant communities in the United States and the sending communities in their home countries because of this knowledge. Many talked about using their expertise to "help" or "give back" to their communities and family members through medical advice.

A few of the nurses were involved in cancer advocacy and awareness in their immigrant communities. For instance, Lara chaired a group bringing breast cancer awareness and education to the Nigerian immigrant community in the DC area. She worked actively to urge her coethnics to go for routine breast exams and mammograms. Her advocacy, which also included several fundraising events a year, was sparked by her own experience as a survivor of the disease. At her invitation, I attended a fundraising walk/run in which scores of women, mostly Nigerian, in running shorts and white t-shirts with the logo of their nursing professional organization and breast cancer pink ribbons, participated. I also attended a swanky fundraising dinner held at a high-end resort and convention center in suburban Maryland attended mostly by Nigerian nurses, physicians, occupational therapists, and other health care professionals.

Similarly, Helen, an oncology nurse, was involved in breast cancer work in her home country of Sierra Leone and donated monies to an organization working there. Other nurses worked through their churches to travel and volunteer their service in not just their own countries but also in other developing countries, through short-term church "mission trips." West African immigrant women health care professionals had formed vibrant organizations, such as the African Women's Cancer Awareness Association (AWCAA), an organization established in 2004 with the stated mission to "work to reduce the burden of cancer on African immigrant women and their families by providing equal access to screening and care for all African women in the US and abroad."[11] The AWCAA also had organized "medical missions" to several African countries, including Nigeria, Sierra Leone, Cameroon, and Sudan. Individual nurses also were part of professional organizations, such as the Northern America Ghana Nurses Foundation, the National Association of Nigerian Nurses in North America, and other local associations, where they engaged in fundraising and health drives, including activities like free diabetes and blood pressure screening and efforts to mobilize their communities to adopt healthy lifestyles. While such efforts were personally meaningful and provided tremendous intrinsic satisfaction, their collective activism was clearly tied to their professional identities as health care workers.

In response to questions about the future, several health care workers talked about returning to their home countries permanently to "give back." For many, the plans were vague and aspirational. For example, they said simply that they hoped to "retire back home." However, a few spoke in concrete and passionate terms about desires to return home to contribute their biomedical expertise and knowledge, and to help alleviate the problems of poor health care infrastructures, "brain drain," low professional morale, and lack of resources that they believed plagued the health care systems of the sending countries. Here, again, intrinsic and extrinsic rewards combined. Many said they wanted to "help others back home," but some saw it as a way to advance their own careers, or to move on to the next stage of their personal and professional lives, as well. They hoped to parlay their U.S.-honed knowledge, expertise, and experience into well-paying and prestigious roles in the government or an international aid bureaucracy.

Helen already had applied for a job with the United Nations. As she explained: "One of my long-term goals would be to help. . . . To go back [to Sierra Leone] if I'm able to do it and help third world countries and focus on young women with breast cancer." Arthurlina also said: "I don't really mind going back [home to Sierra Leone] and assisting with teaching at the university level. I wouldn't mind going back to teach, but also maybe, going back and launching a health care center and trying to make a difference in people's lives." These amorphous dreams nonetheless reflected a mélange of prosocial and extrinsic motivations. Albert, the Sierra Leonean QIDP, had obtained a master's degree in public health while working at Worldwide. He planned to pursue a PhD in the same field. He also talked about returning to Sierra Leone—to enter politics. His goal was to become minister of health. He spoke passionately about using the knowledge he had amassed in the United States to craft policy and provide leadership that would help improve the conditions for individuals with intellectual and physical disabilities in that country. It is not clear whether any of the other care workers would actualize their goals of "return," and the literature on return migration among West African professionals is still nascent. In any case, the belief that they had tangible skills, knowledge, and resources to contribute to their home countries differentiated them from the low-wage home care workers studied by Coe, who were defeated and deflated after their years of service in America.

STRIVING TOWARD THE AMERICAN DREAM

West African immigrant care workers like Helen, Arthurlina, and Albert may have made tangible and intangible gains through their work in the United States, even enough to motivate their aspirations to "give back" to their home countries. But have they achieved the American dream? If so, is their American dream true to the traditional and mythical "rags to riches" depiction popularized by Horatio Alger? If the American dream is measured in professional mobility, educational attainment, entrepreneurship, and stark materialism, then, in making a pathway to professional success and in buying homes in suburban neighborhoods and opening businesses in health care, some West Africans have come close to the American dream. We have seen, however, that the material and professional gains made by nurses came at a huge cost to quality of life and through work in stressful and difficult conditions. While gaining professional satisfaction and intrinsic rewards, it is doubtful that the disability professionals have had commensurate financial success. Even though African immigrants have made inroads in opening businesses in the Washington, DC, metropolitan area, they have not come to dominate the health care industry nationally, like other ethnic businesses such as the Indian moteliers studied by sociologist Pawan Dhingra. Dhingra reported that Indian immigrant motel owners "have created what likely is the largest ethnic enterprise in U.S. history. They claim about half of all the nations motels and hotels, with a concentration in lower- and middle budget motels" (Dhingra 2012, 1). African immigrant-owned health care businesses have not built considerable wealth that will be the launching pad for the next generation. As shown in chapter 3, some of the home health and disability support businesses opened by West Africans were small-scale operations, with indications that many fail, or they are in their infancy and have simply not yet stood the test of time. Worldwide, a successful business launched by Sierra Leonean immigrants, with major clout in the local disability support and administration bureaucracy, and which had integrated the second-generation children of the company founders, was a notable exception.

Indeed, the achievements of the children of immigrants, as refracted through the cultural frames of their immigrant communities and the host society, have become a litmus test for the success of migration projects (Estrada 2019; Louie 2012; Smith 2006; Suárez Orozco and Suárez Orozco 1995). Notably, sociologist Robert Smith articulated the concept of the "immigrant bargain," which accounts for parents' sacrifices in moving to a new country, sometimes to improve children's educational opportunities and professional success. The immigrant bargain serves as a heuristic device to explain the expectation that children work hard to repay their parents' sacrifices, by helping their parents financially and/or making them proud through their achievements.[12] Other scholars have argued that parents' "cultural frame of reference" shapes what success means for immigrant parents and their children. For instance, in her study of the Nigerian immigrant second genera-tion in Britain and the United States, sociologist Onoso Imoagene found they possessed a "success frame," using the concept developed by sociologists Jenni-fer Lee and Min Zhou. In this frame, first-generation Nigerian immigrants who are generally hyper-selected[13] in terms of premigration human, social, and cul-tural capital had inculcated in their children "the expectation . . . that the children, the second generation, had to complete college" (Imoagene 2017, 79). In fact, the cultural norm of obtaining not just undergraduate degrees but pro-fessional degrees in medicine, law, engineering, etc., was internalized by these children of immigrants as an intrinsic part of what it "means to be Nigerian." The framing of success as part of a particularly Nigerian immigrant cultural ethos was reflected in this statement by one of Imoagene's respondents: "It was un-Nigerian not to go to college." Other studies of West African immigrant communities have noted a similar valorization of education and a cultural ethos of viewing education as the pathway to success among Nigerian and other national groups (Halter and Showers Johnson 2014). Indeed, there is evidence that the West African immigrant second generation are overrepresented among Black admis-sions to selective colleges, and that second-generation Nigerian and Ghanaians were the mostly likely among African-origin youth to enter selective universities (Bennett and Lutz 2009; Massey et al. 2007). However, in her account, Imo-agene clarified that it was not "culture" alone that was responsible for Nigerian success. She also showed how structural factors, including immigrant selectivity, the context of reception (including the fact that the second generation were ben-eficiaries of affirmative action policies as they relate to education), social capital generated within the ethnic networks (e.g., tutoring groups within the Nigerian immigrant community that augmented public school educations), etc., all facili-tated the educational and professional achievements of the children of Nigerian immigrants.

I found clear evidence of a similar "success frame" only among a few West African immigrant health care workers. Lara spoke proudly of her twin daughters, who were away at college. As it happened, they attended the university where I was enrolled as a graduate student at the time, and Lara was quite excited by this. It helped build rapport between us, and she spoke proudly of her daughters' accomplishments majoring in science fields. She expected her daughters would go on to become physicians. Others, especially the Sierra Leoneans, took pride in my enrollment in a doctoral program. For example, a Sierra Leonean nurse introduced me to her young children with the statement, "You see, Auntie is going to be a doctor." Other research participants had children completing high school when I met them. In those encounters, they appeared eager to engage with someone associated with a U.S. university, and I helped answer general questions about the college application process. These parents did not strike me, however, as very knowledgeable about college admissions, nor did they seem to have clear ideas about what their children should do to be successful in their college applications, and in life, in the way that has been depicted as typical in the cultural norms of American middle-class parenthood (Lareau 2003) or upper middle-class professional, Nigerians (Imoagene 2017).

As described in chapter 2, health care workers actively urged their children and young relatives to enter entry-level health care fields, and in some cases, these care pioneers urged them to eschew other college majors and career paths. Several interviewees revealed that their U.S.-born or raised children already were located in the health care field. Most were studying to become nurses or training in other allied health sciences, such as to become physician assistants, while working as home health aides or nursing aides. I also met U.S.-born West African job applicants and new DSP trainees at Worldwide. Lara was thus unusual among the health care workers I met in envisioning that her children would become doctors.

The views of parents regarding their children's prospects within health care was captured in a statement made by Anwar, a Sierra Leonean administrator of a home health agency: "I'll be happy if my eldest daughter who is now in school [becomes a nurse]. She was trying to do LPN. I'm going to encourage her to do more." Other parents also actively encouraged their children to study nursing. There was only one nurse who stated emphatically that she did not want her child to become a nurse, based on her own experience with nursing. Not only did Nurse X not want her daughter to go into nursing, but she also admitted that had she herself been born in America she didn't think she would have been a nurse. She stated: "So, I think [nursing] is the best thing for my situation since I'm an African, because of my accent. But if I was born in America . . . Like my daughter, I told her (I have a daughter that's in college), I told her 'I don't want you to be a nurse, it's not easy.'" Given this conversation, I was surprised when she later revealed that her daughter was planning for a future in health care and studying to be a physician's assistant.

Those immigrants who arrived as children, as well as the children of immigrants that I met, for the most part were ambivalent to enter the field themselves. As Jennifer, a Nigerian nurse practitioner put it, "I did not want to be yet another African nurse." Yet, she and her brother followed their mother and five aunts into nursing. Such cases raise some questions: What forces caused these American-born or raised-American young people to enter the field? And what does their decision-making processes and prospects tell us about the limits of the American dream?

INHERITING A LABOR NICHE: THE AFRICAN IMMIGRANT 1.5 AND SECOND GENERATION

In addition to the immigrant family networks described in chapter 2, young American-born or raised-American nurses, like their first-generation counterparts, sometimes became nurses because of blocked opportunities in the U.S. labor market or after facing personal and professional setbacks. In some cases, they had obtained bachelor's degrees in other fields (e.g., business administration) but switched to nursing degrees after struggling to find work or after being laid off from previous jobs. The case of Sade, a director of nursing in a West African-owned home health care business, is instructive. Born in the United States to Nigerian immigrant parents, she returned to Nigeria with her parents when she was very young. When she was twelve, her mother moved back to the United States with Sade and her older sister. Her older sister later studied nursing. Sade graduated from a state university with a bachelor's degree in business administration, refusing her older sister's urging that she also study nursing. Later, Sade would come to regret that decision, as she said: "But I just got laid off so many times that I'm like, no matter what, my sister, she would always have her job . . . And at that point that I also got laid off, I was a single mother. So, I needed to go and do something. So, I didn't go into it [nursing] initially because I love the blood and the taking care of people and all that. I really went there initially for job security."

Other 1.5-generation research participants told similar stories of blocked opportunities or unfilled professional goals. For example, Jennifer, who didn't want to be "yet another African nurse," wanted to major in computer science in college, but "it was too hard." Then, after not getting accepted into pharmacy school, she started training to be a nurse. She described coming to that decision thus: "I guess I was meant to do it because everything else kind of didn't work out, so it's like, OK, you know. I took it that way, so it's like, OK, maybe I was meant to be a nurse." Sade, the second-generation nurse manager at a West African owned agency, aside from being "laid off from jobs," reported that she had "had trouble with the law" in her young adulthood. A criminal record, therefore, limited her opportunity in the primary labor market and explained her decision to work within the West African labor niche.

Others framed their decisions to enter nursing by highlighting the financial rewards of the job or, like Sade, the job security. Yvonne, a master's-degreed nurse from Liberia who had arrived in the United States at age five, held the title Immunization Compliance Nurse for a major school district. She described herself as a "glorified school nurse." She described her decision to enter the profession thus:

> Well, I think, probably me seeing my mother, because I saw her go to school and try to be a nurse. But to be quite honest too, I kind of always been the type of person who likes to play it safe, and I did not want to have a career where I would have difficulty in finding positions or making money. And I know that may sound like that's not why you should take a career path but also, I had seen . . . also my mother's sisters are nurses, aunts, so I had seen it and been accustomed to it so much, that it was probably the only other option.

Yvonne, like the other American-born or raised-American children of West African immigrants, was clearly influenced by care pioneers within West African immigrant ethnic networks. However, her reference to struggles to finding a job, or "making money," speak to the enduring obstacles to reaping the full and undiluted benefits of the American dream for Blacks in America. These obstacles were explored by sociologist Maya Beasley, who described how talented Black undergraduates were steered away from high-paying and high-status careers for fear of anticipated discrimination. Yvonne seems to have this concern, as well. Like their immigrant parents or elders who faced obstacles in the U.S. labor market and entered health care fields, these childhood arrivals and children of immigrants also faced similar problems: personal troubles and failures, "concrete ceilings" (Durr and Wingfield 2011), or the general realization that there were few options available to them. For these new Americans, health care fields seem like a safe bet in a society in which opportunities remain stratified by race. Immigrant parents, as care pioneers whose own initiation into the labor market was through health care professions and whose frame of reference for success in America was largely limited to professional health care fields, actively steered their children and young relatives into this field.

Not all children of West African immigrant health care workers become health care workers themselves, and not all health care workers want their children to follow their path. However, my observations suggest that the 1.5 and second generation of West African immigrants are entering the health care labor niche populated by the first generation and oftentimes work alongside their first-generation counterparts. In doing so, they belie some of the assumptions around immigration, particularly upward mobility and the American dream. Discussing these issues in relation to immigrant entrepreneurs, sociologist Pawan Dhingra writes: "The standard assumption has been that the grandchildren, if not the children, of immigrant business owners will move into the standard labor market as they become college educated and more job opportunities present themselves" (Dhingra 2012, 81).

This was the case of the European migrants of the early twentieth century, and more recently, this assumption holds true for Korean, Chinese, Vietnamese, and some Indian groups, whose children moved out of the ethnic enclave economy and integrated into professional and white-collar jobs. By moving out of the businesses occupied by their immigrant parents, which they view as "too small and too low status" (Dhingra 2012, 81), these second-generation immigrants are fulfilling the "immigrant bargain." The parents actively encouraged their children to move out of these "ethnic niches" of employment. Dae Young Kim (2006) described how Korean immigrants encouraged their children to choose "safe professions" such as medicine or law. They saw these professions as protective shields against racism as well as penury. By contrast, my research shows the African immigrant 1.5 and second generations moving into the ethnic niche populated by the first generation, often with the encouragement of the pioneering generation. This may be, in part, due to the intractable nature of anti-Black racism in the United States, which may make parents less optimistic that the right credentials can protect their children from facing constrained opportunities. It also may reflect the fact that the African immigrants I interviewed, in contrast to some of the Asian groups others have studied, were not working in an enclave economy, catering to coethnics, or as "middle-man" minorities catering exclusively to U.S. minority groups. Instead, they were working in mainstream private or government institutions or government-sponsored businesses largely funded through federal and state funding streams (Medicaid) catering to diverse groups of service recipients. Work in the primary labor market and in institutional health care may be perceived as higher status than work in the ethnic enclave economy or secondary markets.

Immigrants of the 1.5 and second generation were, however, more likely to capitalize on previous educational credentials and experiences or take their nursing degrees to "the next level" than their parents or elders. For instance, Jennifer was a nurse practitioner, Yvonne held a master's degree in public health and an MBA in addition to her nursing degree, and Sade brought her bachelor's degree in business to bear by going into health care staffing and administration. They were more likely to strategically deploy these credentials to move out of bedside care than the first generation. Just as they had credited their immigrant parents and coethnics for their decision to enter nursing, some in this group learned from these care pioneers' experiences in the field. They used these lessons to circumvent the more negative parts of the profession and to maximize the professional rewards. For instance, Jennifer explained: "Well, I knew that when I first started working on the floor [of the hospital], what really made me go back to school was my mother, because she works in a maternity unit] and she also works in a telemetry unit [meaning she works two jobs]. So I see how hard she works. She works the night shift, she works day shift, and then when I started working as a nurse, then I'm like, oh, this is hard work. I just couldn't see myself doing that in my 50s at all."

Sociologist Emir Estrada, who studied Latinx immigrant street vendors in Los Angeles, noted that parents working alongside their children hoped their children would understand the difficulties of the job and their lives on the street enough so they would make different educational, career, and life choices. American-raised African immigrants like Jennifer had internalized this lesson. Learning from their parents' experiences in bedside nursing, they were determined to move out of it to avoid overwork and punishing hours.

Much of the existing literature that has shed light on children of immigrants who have entered the niches occupied by their immigrant parents focuses on the children of entrepreneurs who have inherited their parents' businesses (Dhingra 2012; Min 2008). The understanding has been that they did so when they could not access the white-collar labor market or, alternatively, when they made the calculation that the American dream was more attainable by building on the wealth and social capital built by their immigrant parents rather than by laboring in professional corporate jobs. Pawan Dhingra described children of Indian immigrants who left professional jobs because they had experienced racial discrimination or felt pigeonholed into technical as opposed to managerial and leadership roles. It is possible that the children of West African immigrants who have set up home care and disability support businesses will follow a similar path. However, unlike the professionals Dhingra describes, they have not even entered other professions as a first step. Instead, they are entering health care occupations, often in the least prestigious and poorest paying jobs, as the first generation did.

CONCLUSION

Arthurlina Stevens, the passionate "real" nurse for whom nursing was a "calling," committed to the profession even as the rewards of her career choice seemed miniscule in her homeland of Sierra Leone. Leaving Sierra Leone amid conflict and political instability, she eventually found career success and fulfillment as a director of nursing in a U.S. nursing home. Albert Kamara, the dignified and diligent university lecturer, had hoped to translate his premigration credentials and professional experience in the United States. Forced to give up this dream, he dedicated himself to the care of individuals with various disabilities. Over time, his previous life experiences and expectations seemed like a distant dream. Both were full of the reflective musings that accompany middle age, many of which, in their case, pertained to what they had achieved in the United States. Proud of the lives they had made for themselves, they had begun to look forward to the next and perhaps final phase of their professional lives. Their dreams of that future entailed plans to "give back" to the societies from which they had come. Albert hoped to enter a career in politics and aspired to become minister of health in Sierra Leone. Arthurlina hoped to return and teach at the university level and to open a clinic. Rose Asamoah was at an earlier stage of life, and she had turned to nursing when other professional ambitions failed. Reflecting, perhaps, her stage in the life cycle, she was focused on her professional life in the United States. She had successfully made the pivot from dreams of being a medical doctor set for her by her parents in Ghana to reaching the pinnacle of her bedside nursing career as a nurse practitioner. She was deciding whether to enroll in a doctorate program in nursing practice at a prestigious U.S. university.

Through stories like those of Arthurlina, Albert, and Rose, this book has shed light on the experiences of West African immigrants, a group that has been largely invisible in scholarly discussions of professional care occupations. Rather than focus on the constraints and challenges of the field, or their exploitation, marginalization, and servitude in certain segments, this book has elucidated the processes that transform immigrants into health care workers. This is not a story that starts in the destination country, and it is not just a story about how a group entered the United States and eventually found their place in the complicated and sometimes sharp-edged mosaic that is multiracial, multicultural U.S. society after a period of struggle. Rather, this book has traced this group's premigration backgrounds, shedding light on the contexts from which they derive, what brought them to the United States, what they brought with them, and how ties with others back home and *care pioneers* where they settled helped explain the path they trod.

This story incorporated multiple scales of analysis, from the aerial view of structure and political economy to the grounds-up view of ethnography. It has illuminated factors at work in the global economy, structural conditions in the sending countries, the role of immigration and labor policies and practices in the United States, and the agency of immigrants themselves, in creating the terms that have incorporated West Africans into various sectors of the U.S. health care industry. This book has traced the big picture of migration and care work while also narrowing in on the lived experiences of individual immigrants, showing how they navigate the challenges of their jobs but also how many come to a place of joy and form identities that are meaningful and rewarding.

Previous scholarship has shed light on the growing demand for health care workers in advanced industrialized countries with aging populations and shortages of professional and paraprofessional care workers. The extant literature on the international recruitment of professional health care workers (nurses, in particular) has focused on structures and agents in sending countries, intermediate actors such as transnational recruitment agencies, and contexts of reception in receiving states, but not on a sustained analysis of immigrant communities and immigrant ethnic networks in creating this labor supply. Some work on paraprofessional health care workers in the United States has noted the concentrations of immigrant women of color and their experiences of work but has not elaborated in depth on the systematic processes that transform immigrants into care workers. Bringing insights from U.S. immigration scholarship to bear, I have drawn attention to the role of formal and informal social networks formed by West Africans as well as their entrepreneurial initiatives around the provision of care. This study has thus shed light upon meso-level actors that tap into a reservoir of immigrant labor to create health care workers in destination countries.

By investigating West African social networks and formal businesses embedded in ethnic networks, and their role in shaping the labor market experiences of West African immigrant health care workers, *Migrants Who Care* has added to the body of knowledge on the creation of ethnic niches of employment in United States immigration. The home care and disability support businesses set up by West African immigrant entrepreneurs in Washington, DC, set them apart from Caribbean immigrants to the United States who generally have been the Black immigrant group that has received a lot of scholarly attention. Existing literature has drawn our attention to the concentrations of English-speaking Caribbean immigrants as domestic and long-term care workers (predominantly as nannies and paraprofessional nursing assistants) in New York City (Carty 2003; Colen 1989, 1990; Vickerman 1999; Foner 1987; Kasinitiz and Vickerman 2001). This literature has done a lot to advance our understanding of their experiences as direct care workers but has not captured a similar experience of Caribbean immigrants as entrepreneurs or business owners in care. This book, in contrast, has illuminated the entrepreneurial activities of West African immigrants who are creating an employment niche in disability support and home care in an industry that is highly regulated by state licensing and governing procedures. The businesses set up by West African immigrants in metropolitan Washington, DC, drew from federal and local government subsidies to hire coethnics and served a predominantly minority, native-born population (African Americans). Unlike other immigrant "middleman minority" entrepreneurs, they operated within the primary labor market and have drawn largely from government funding streams rather than on private capital. This book has brought to light the little-known story of Black African immigrants who have provided long-term care services to underserved U.S. racial minority populations and staffed the occupational segments in professional health care that are the least desired and offer the lowest rewards.

A traditional American framing would suggest that the story told in this book is an immigrant success story. But telling this story as one of grit and gumption, and then triumph, would obscure the systematic processes and structures through which individual women and men, highly skilled and trained in their home countries, became produced, repackaged, and deployed as entry-level health care workers. In the pages of this book, I have named such processes: globalization and labor displacement; wars, political instability, economic insecurity, and the impact of neoliberal economic policies in sending countries; corruption, mismanagement, and the failures of the neocolonial African state; and demographic changes and other socioeconomic processes in the destination country, including neoliberalism, privatization, the retrenchment of U.S. welfare, and the deinstitutionalization of care. An immigrant success story that focuses on the endpoint of a migratory journey also obscures the costs and challenges individuals encountered along the way. Even the most successful individuals I interviewed for this book had made huge, irreversible sacrifices. The Johnsons, for instance, who have achieved a thriving family business and whose family bonds, fortified by the company they have built, seem extremely tight, must have lost something when the parents could not care for their oldest child in her most tender years.

If this book is not the traditional immigrant success story, it is not a story about the exploitation of an immigrant group, either. Not only is a reductive analysis that centers only their location in the global economy and the ways in which they were acted upon by global capitalism incomplete, it would do a grave injustice to the people who entrusted their stories to my care. They did not see themselves as victims. Moving across various analytical vantage points helped me come to what I hope is a nuanced understanding of the terms of their incorporation into the U.S. economy. While a macro-structural approach led me to an indictment of the forces of global capitalism and the institutions of the state, including labor, educational, and credentialing regimes in labor displacement, an investigation of immigrant communities and recruitment practices at the meso-level also led me to the ways that West African immigrant communities created and deployed social capital to capitalize on a segment of the labor market in which there was a structural need. The micro-level analysis also showed how individuals navigated difficult personal and professional circumstances and found pathways to upward mobility.

The micro-level focus on individual subjectivities, identities, and meaning making helped illuminate my understanding of immigrant labor in care work. I showed the processes—physical/embodied and emotional—through which these immigrants became transformed into professional care workers. By an honest discussion of their motivations for entry into care occupations, the initial distress and displacement care workers experienced, and their account of what they gained from their close and intimate caring for others, I have forged an intervention into our understanding of the motivations and rewards of care work. While many are drawn into care occupations because of intrinsic, altruistic, and prosocial motivations, and gain intrinsic rewards even in the absence of material and extrinsic rewards (Stacey 2005, 2011), we can begin to understand and acknowledge that this is not always the case, all the time. Most of the individuals in this book went into care occupations with far from noble or altruistic motivations. But in focusing on how immigrants are produced, repackaged, and deployed as care workers, I have sought to expand our understanding of the structural forces that compel newcomers to the United States to become care workers, what factors help them stay in their jobs, and under what circumstances they are able to move onward and upward and across professional segments.

The case of West African immigrants shows that intrinsic and extrinsic motivations and rewards may not necessarily be mutually exclusive. People may enter these occupations for a host of reasons and may gain a combination of rewards. The practical implications are worth underscoring. These occupations draw from those who are "called" to care, including those who may have previously cared for loved ones, as well as people with very few options elsewhere in the labor market, people who can envisage a stepwise career progression from direct care work to professional positions in nursing, for instance, or those seeking a secure and "recession proof" path to economic security. Such understandings of motivations can help us reframe the way we think about care occupations and the way we reward those who enter them. Focusing on these various motivations for entry also can help us create more typologies and nuanced distinctions among various occupational categories in care work. For instance, nursing can align with the motivations of financial rewards and job security, as opposed to domestic cleaners and home health aides who may be compelled to care for lack of other options in the labor market. This book also has supported a major argument advocated by care work scholars, which is that, regardless of the motivations for entry, care work, with its deep and close affective and emotional as well as physical connections between workers and care recipients, does have the power to transform those who engage in it. If there was one thing that all the persons I met had in common, it was that they all acknowledged that their location and experiences in health care work had irrevocably transformed them.

This book also has shed light on the workings of race, gender, and ethnicity in health care institutions. I found support for existing claims about the prevalence and persistence of racism in nursing and for the understanding of health care institutions as racialized and gendered organizations (Wingfield 2009, 2019; Wingfield and Chavez 2020). To that existing body of knowledge, I have added an understanding of how ethnicity, nativity status, and work contexts shape the reception and experience of health workers. I also outlined a particular form of racial animus toward Africans, *African-origin discrimination*, and the perception among African care workers that they occupied the bottom of racially stratified hierarchies in mainstream health care institutions. The findings solidified the intersections of race, gender, ethnicity, and nativity status in shaping the experiences of individual workers, but also have wider implications for our understanding of race and immigration in the United States. Rather than presenting Black immigrants as a monolith, I have argued for the heterogeneity of experience among different Black immigrant groups. I showed how ethnicity, stereotypes, and meanings associated with regional or national origin shaped the reception of Africans in ways that were divergent from what scholars have identified among English-speaking Caribbean groups. I identified the strategies West African immigrants used to resist racism, combat racial stereotypes, and navigate structural barriers in nursing. Through the concept of *professional distancing*, I have illuminated a particular strategy deployed by some West African immigrant nurses to seek upward mobility in nursing. I also showed the limits of this and other individual-level strategies in upending structural and institutionalized racial hierarchies.

I have shown that, contrary to some assumptions in the care work literature, entry-level care occupations and direct care work need not lead to professional dead ends. I have traced a pathway of mobility among West African immigrants from direct care work to professional nursing or positions of authority in disability support. I acknowledge that this path requires tremendous amounts of social capital. The overwhelming majority of participants, in addition to possessing premigration class privilege, benefitted from social capital embedded within their immigrant ethnic networks as well as transnational social capital. I have shown how already-established West African immigrants initiated the migration of others and helped absorb the cost of settlement, making the professional mobility of later arrivals that much more possible. While many sent financial remittances back home, much like the West African immigrants Faranak Miraftab studied, the flow of resources was far from unidirectional. Many relied on family members who remained in the home country for help with childcare, either through leaving young children behind as they embarked on their journeys or, as in the case of the Johnsons and a couple of others I met, by sending their U.S.-born children to the home country to save on childcare costs. This outsourcing of reproductive labor afforded these immigrants the time to earn and save more and to develop their human capital, which then solidified their steps as they climbed up the professional ladder.

The upward mobility traced in this story should be celebrated and applauded. At the same time, the view of the nursing profession as a pathway to economic prosperity that has circulated in West African immigrant networks raises serious concern. Many study participants who were lured into nursing by the promises of success they heard from or saw in others reported job satisfaction, fulfillment, and growth. They also reported genuine concern for the well-being of their patients. Some used their expertise to engage in health advocacy and service in their communities. However, the pressure to go into nursing "for the money," as many said, and the long hours and other strategies deployed to reach financial goals raise serious concerns regarding effective clinical practice, ethical practice, and the well-being of patients. Participants experienced strong pressure to gain further credentials and move up from direct care work to credentialed nursing. They embarked on protracted educational journeys filled with fits and starts as they balanced work and education. The financial pressures to afford tuition costs led to enrollment in the most affordable and accessible educational institutions. This raises concern about the quality of training, the legitimacy of credentials earned, and the potential for unscrupulous elements to traffic in an illicit market for these coveted credentials. Indeed, as of this writing, there are allegations of such a market in Maryland.[1] Future research might address these questions more directly through observations of care. We must celebrate those who took the path of mobility in health care and applaud those who are fully committed to the well-being of others. However, we must question the global, structural, and institutional arrangements that make it so that some immigrants feel compelled to care.

This case study on West African immigrants has some policy and practical implications for direct care work and the nursing profession. Many of the prescriptions I will soon discuss have been noted by other scholars and may be currently in practice in some institutions. These practices should be expanded and implemented more widely. The stepwise path that some participants took from direct care work to credentialed nursing supports the argument that other scholars have made that there should be career lattices and ladders within nursing education and paraprofessional health care professions (Buch 2018; Coe 2019). These lattices would ensure that nursing aides could advance to positions of greater seniority, skill, and authority in a stepwise fashion, earning credentials and incremental higher pay and responsibility along the way. These ladders also should respect and honor work experience across segments. For example, DSP and HHA experience could, under some circumstances, transfer over into nursing.

Health care institutions such as nursing homes and hospitals that have experienced staffing shortages and challenges could provide grants and financial subsidies toward further education for current certified nursing assistants and other direct care workers to earn further credentials, with the stipulation that they remain in employment for an agreed-upon length of time. Educational institutions also could do more to recruit students among underrepresented populations and in underserved communities and provide them with financial aid and support.

Beyond these measures for career advancement, as many others have argued, building a stable direct care workforce that will meet current and projected needs means that workers should be guaranteed a living wage and adequate benefits, including health care (see, for example, Stacey 2011). Other practical solutions, such as transportation vouchers, childcare cost reimbursements, and paid sick leave would help attract a committed and skilled labor force and work toward retaining them (see, for example, Cranford 2020; Schweid 2021). As the COVID-19 pandemic has laid bare, direct care workers such as nursing assistants and home care workers were particularly vulnerable to infection, as were residents in congregate settings such as nursing homes. These interlocking systems of interdependence and vulnerability amplify the calls for urgent reform of U.S. long-term care. In the COVID-19 era, there is an urgent need to provide adequate compensation so that home care workers and nursing aides are not forced to work multiple jobs or with multiple patients, increasing the risk of infection to themselves and their charges. Paraprofessional health care workers should be valued and respected and provided with adequate support, including sufficient access to personal protective equipment in the COVID-19 era and adequate supplies and tools beyond the pandemic.

This book also has implications for the training of paraprofessional care workers. The experience of disability support professionals showed there were gaps between training provided by agencies as mandated by state oversight bodies and the actual needs of care receivers. Interview and observation data as well as my personal experience with the online training for DSP certification suggest the trainings were designed to impart technical and medicalized knowledge and to emphasize policies and ethical concerns. Much effort was placed on measures to protect the safety, bodily integrity, and dignity of the persons needing care. It is certainly essential that care workers understand at the level of theory the special needs of vulnerable populations of care recipients. However, as anthropologist Elana Buch has argued, in addition to these technical and didactic materials, there must be "ongoing opportunities to explore the moral, relational, and emotional complexities of home care work [and disability support/nursing assistance]" (Buch 2018, 212). As this research has illuminated, many care workers were unprepared to deal with the emotional and relational aspects of care. Buch and others also have argued for recognizing and rewarding care workers with longevity of service and experience. I also would propose that opportunities for more formalized mentorship systems, such as preceptorships, should be built in. More experienced care workers should be paired with new recruits so they can pass on the experiential part of training. Disability support professionals who feel unprepared for the actual work of care after existing orientation might benefit from such a mentorship system. This study also suggests the need for opportunities for ongoing training on patient-provider communication, including cross-cultural communication for both care receivers and care recipients in home care. Such trainings, in which foreign-born care workers are oriented to the needs of U.S. care recipients, including traditions around food, religious expectations, language diversity, etc., are important. For their own part, care recipients must be encouraged to acknowledge and respect the backgrounds and diversity of care staff. As many have argued, direct care workers need to be valued and integrated as full-fledged members of care teams with input in the decision-making processes as they relate to individualized support and care plans, etc. (see, for example, Dodson and Zincavage 2015).

This study reinforces the arguments about racism and racial stratification in the nursing profession. Health care institutions should do more to address racial inequities in organizational structures, including racialized hierarchies in specializations, underrepresentation of minorities in positions of authority, and racial barriers to credentialing, shift allocation, etc. Racial bias, stereotyping, microaggressions, and discrimination at the interpersonal level should be addressed with consequences such as dismissal, suspension, and official reprimands for individual perpetrators. There should be policies to address systemic and interpersonal racism in health care institutions beyond diversity initiatives and cultural competency training. These policies and strategies to target racial inequities should begin with nursing education. There should be a greater emphasis on social determinants of health and racial disparities in health in nursing school curricular. Instructors and students must be made more aware of the robust literature regarding racism in nursing schools and institutions, and racism in provider-patient interactions. Incorporating these social perspectives more centrally into nursing education might work toward changing climates and cultures that will transfer from nursing classrooms to the hallways of hospitals, clinics, doctor's offices, and nursing homes.

Migrants Who Care also has important lessons and takeaways for policymakers in both the sending and receiving societies. Much has been made of the "brain drain" of skilled professionals in Africa and other areas of the developing world: scientists, doctors, professors, civil servants, and nurses who leave because of failures of institutions and the state to retain them. And there is a robust literature on the "brain drain" of professional health care workers. Others have noted the failure to translate those skills and resources into commensurate positions in the receiving nations, leading to what some have termed "brain waste" (see for example, Gwaradzimba and Shumba 2010; Zeleza 2009). Others describe the same phenomena as the "de-skilling" of immigrant workers. Certainly, some of the voices we heard in this book expressed the pain and frustration of loss of intellectual resources and human capital. However, this book joins others that have elucidated another phenomenon situated between "brain drain" and "brain waste": how talented individuals retrain and develop drastically new skills that make them marketable, even invaluable, to the labor markets of host societies. This book has identified a group of trained health care workers who are not captured in the "brain drain" of the health care worker narrative. These are individuals who had developed their human capital in other areas in sending countries but became "re-skilled" as health care workers upon migration. West African nations, many of which suffer the devastating effects of crumbling health care infrastructures, should put more effort into harnessing the skills and resources of these workers. Study participants already volunteer their expertise on a temporary basis, and some aspire to contribute their proficiencies to their homelands permanently. Governments and nongovernmental organizations would do well to encourage the circulation of skills and resources. For instance, members of the West African health care work diaspora could be encouraged to return for moderately funded "sabbaticals," where they could collaborate with their counterparts in sharing resources, knowledge, and expertise. This study suggests that the diasporic health care workers would welcome the opportunity to "give back," and such a scheme would build the capacity of institutions and workers in the home countries.

The successful pathways of the individuals profiled in this book were ultimately made possible by their legal immigration status in the United States, via the diversity visa lottery, family reunification, employment, and refugee provisions in immigration law. Access to legal status or "papers" turned migrant dreams into realities. And contrary to anti-immigration rhetoric and policy, these immigrants were working hard at some of the most undesired and undesirable jobs. Millions of immigrants work under similar circumstances every day, many of them under the chronic threat of deportation. We can truly live in a caring society when we value those who care for our sick, our elders, our children; those who grow our food; those who clean bodies and bowel movements, as well as our homes and offices and afford them and the vulnerable among us not only legal protection but basic human decency.

AFTERWORD

COVID-19

I collected the data for this book well before the COVID-19 pandemic began in March 2020 but wrote much of it in that turbulent time. Throughout, I was conscious that the subjects of the book had become central players as "frontline" or "essential workers" in the fight against this deadly disease, a fact which has undoubtedly had implications for the story I have told in this book.

In the early days of the outbreak, the media hailed "frontline" health care workers as "heroes" in the fight against the virus. These "heroes" were typically imagined and depicted as doctors and professional staff within hospitals, not home health aides, certified nursing assistants, or direct support staff who care for the vulnerable and disabled people in home or institutional long-term care settings. Immigrant workers, and in particular, Black immigrant workers, were noticeably absent in the discourses of "heroic" frontline health care staff. To the extent that the media turned its attention to care settings beyond hospitals, it was in connection with horrific outbreaks of the virus and deaths of older residents in congregate settings, especially in nursing homes (Chidambaram, Garfield, and Neuman 2020; Freed et al. 2020). Yet, little attention was paid to the workers in these settings, especially low-wage direct care workers. It goes without saying that the experiences of African immigrant care workers in nursing homes and private homes of the most vulnerable was largely ignored.[1]

As I watched these news reports, my thoughts turned to the care workers I had met. How had they fared during the pandemic? What were their experiences within mainstream health care settings, private home environments, and African-owned disability support businesses? How did the pandemic affect existing stratification in nursing, and in health care more broadly? In what ways would the findings of this book help us make sense of inequality among health care workers in various work contexts?

In August 2020, I reconnected with Miriam, the director of nursing at Worldwide, and three registered nurses (two Sierra Leonean and one Nigerian) whom I had interviewed for the book project and with whom I was still in touch. I made informal phone calls to check on them. I asked about their health and how they were doing in general. From August to October 2021, I contacted them again and completed more formal interviews. During this time, I also interviewed three additional Sierra Leonean nurses I had come to know after data collection for the book was complete. Unlike the research subjects for the book, the three additional respondents did not live in the Washington, DC, metropolitan area. The more formal interviews happened more than a year after the original outbreak and after vaccines had become widely available for adult populations. I asked how they were doing at the time, but also asked them to reflect on their experiences between March to May 2020 (the early days) of the pandemic, as well as their experiences during the various peaks of infections and death associated with the virus where they live.

I also followed commentary by African health care workers on social media, news media reports on health care workers, the general emerging social scientific and public health literature on COVID-19, and the writings of colleagues such as anthropologist Cati Coe, who published a short opinion/policy piece from follow-up interviews she had conducted with West African immigrant home care workers between August and October 2020. The information reported in this brief afterword are preliminary thoughts about the impact of COVID-19 on individual West African immigrant health care workers, and addresses some of the themes that were emerging at the time of this book's writing and publication.

As I argued in the book, the context of work and the profile of care recipients together shape the experiences of African immigrant health and direct care workers, including the professional identities they develop and the emotional labor they perform. For instance, disability support professionals working in ethnically owned businesses and caring for intellectually disabled care recipients earned relatively low wages but built on social capital in their ethnic networks to gain professional mobility. They also experienced their emotional labor as rewarding and fulfilling. Nurses in predominantly white settings, on the other hand, found their jobs intrinsically and extrinsically rewarding but navigated tense and hostile climates and negative experiences with patients, supervisors, and co-workers. Likewise, during the COVID-19 pandemic, different care workers had different experiences based on the type of institution or setting in which they worked and their roles within them.

Owners of custodial care businesses, such as the Johnsons, navigated the pandemic as small business owners. They had to make serious decisions and enact protocols to keep their workers and care recipients safe. They also dealt with the financial fallout and costs of the pandemic. Miriam recalled confusion in the early days of the pandemic. Worldwide scrambled to come up with safety protocols and secure personal protective equipment (PPE) for their staff amid miscommunication from the local disability support bureaucracy. Lapses in government leadership at the local level mirrored the chaotic and decentered response to the pandemic in several states and at the federal level (GAO 2020; McGarry et al. 2020; MITRE Corporation 2020; Pradhan et al. 2020). After initially competing with similar businesses to secure PPE with local suppliers on a weekly basis, they used their private connections to a larger supplier in California to secure PPE for their staff long-term. They created a COVID task force comprising the senior leadership at Worldwide to coordinate their response to the pandemic. The task force had virtual weekly meetings throughout the early months of the pandemic, and served as the crisis command center, making decisions to modify company operations.

To prevent the spread of the virus among their care recipients, Worldwide decided to close the day center, which was serving 130 persons at the time, and they focused on residential care. The closure forced them to furlough some of their staff, and a few others, worried about the risk of contagion, left their jobs. Rather than having many staff working twelve-hour shifts as they had done pre-pandemic, they had a key cadre of staff who worked 24/7 in the residential settings on a two-week on, two-week off rotation. As Miriam put it, they asked staff "to sit tight in the homes for two weeks." These measures were meant to mitigate the spread of the virus, and probably did so. Research has shown that care staff who worked multiple shifts with different employers and care recipients not only increased their exposure but were at high risk of spreading the virus (Chapman and Harrington 2020; Coe 2021; Cigler 2021). Preliminary evidence suggests that other African home care workers who worked as live-in elder care workers through private arrangements or via recruitment agencies also protected themselves by staying longer in the home of clients rather than taking breaks to go back to their own homes or being relieved by a different care worker (Coe 2021).

Worldwide ran education campaigns about physical distancing and other public health measures to prevent COVID among their staff and the local community. The COVID-19 task force initiated a system of internal contact tracing and isolation/quarantine measures to mitigate the spread of the virus. They did not return to regular staff schedules until summer 2020, at which point they mandated monthly testing for the coronavirus for every employee. This testing was still ongoing as of summer 2021. When vaccines became available, they took the initiative to administer COVID-19 vaccines to all their staff. They ran vaccine clinics in partnership with a local Walgreens pharmacy. When vaccines became widely available, they mandated that all their existing staff should get vaccines within ninety days and all new employees should do so within thirty days. They reported that about ten staff left their employ because of these mandates. Despite the measures in place, twelve residents and twenty staff were infected, although the last positive test of a staff member was December 2020. There were no resident deaths, but two Worldwide staff members who were in their fifties and sixties died. These mortality and morbidity rates appear remarkably low compared to other care settings. African care workers in congregate settings such as nursing homes had higher rates of infection and they certainly witnessed many resident deaths, as other research shows (Coe 2021).

By summer 2021, Worldwide seemed to have survived the worst of the pandemic. Miriam reported that they had received pandemic-related financial relief for small businesses and had accessed loans from the Payment Protection Program,[2] which helped them survive financially "without going in the red." She reported support from state administrators and bureaucrats in navigating the financial impact. For instance, DDS had updated their billing codes and processes to cover employee overtime and the costs of PPE. Miriam told me she doubted that smaller African-owned businesses would survive the pandemic in the long run. She also spoke about the toll of the pandemic on the African immigrant community in the area overall. "Everyone knew someone who had died," she said. Ms. Aisha Deen, a well-known registered nurse in the area, and a devoted member of the African Women's Cancer Awareness Association[3] who volunteered her services through that organization, was one loss that seemed to be communally shared.

The experiences of the staff, residents, and administrators at Worldwide reflect the larger themes on COVID-19 reported in the media. They provide a worm's eye view of the impact on under-resourced segments of the health and long-term care industries. For example, the shortage of PPE for essential workers early in the pandemic put direct care workers at risk of contracting the virus and potentially spreading to vulnerable care recipients. Exposure to the virus, lack of adequate PPE, job insecurity as families scaled back paid care for vulnerable older adults, stress, burnout, fatigue, and infection affected many direct care workers in homes and institutional settings (Coe 2021; Chapman and Harrington 2020; Cigler 2021; Van Houtven et al. 2020.

Worldwide showed exceptional leadership and resourcefulness in combating the virus and protecting their residents and staff. While much attention in media and academic circles has been drawn to the impact of the pandemic on large institutions, such as nursing homes and hospitals, the impact on care recipients and workers in smaller-size residential care homes, such as group homes, small day programs, and private home settings, is worth exploring further in the coming years.

Nurses' experiences of the pandemic also varied by type of institution in which they worked and their roles within them. Helen, a Sierra Leonean oncology nurse and a key informant for this book, had become an administrator in a prestigious research and teaching hospital attached to a prestigious university when I caught up with her during the pandemic. She confronted the pandemic as a leader responsible for staff safety and patient welfare, broadly defined. As a nurse manager of an outpatient oncology clinic, she did not treat COVID patients but could speak in detail about the effect on her predominantly white colleagues in her unit and the nursing profession in general. She was a part of

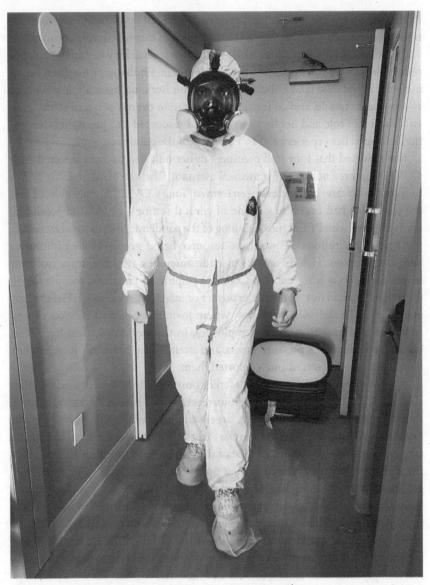

FIGURE A.1. A nurse working on the frontlines of COVID-19. (Photo courtesy Joseph Cole, RN.)

decision-making teams responsible for crafting new protocols, policies, and safety guidelines as her unit carried on with non-COVID-related care. She reported increased workload for the administrative staff as they created new operating procedures for the COVID environment but cuts to clinical staff because of reduced in-person operations at the beginning of the pandemic. She reflected on the financial impact on furloughed workers, especially on lower-wage medical assistants.

At the same time, she felt the pandemic had provided opportunities for innovation in telemedicine, as they shifted to that mode of care for routine consultation with patients. In my discussion with Helen, I was struck by her analytical and reflective take on the impact of the pandemic in a holistic rather than on an individual level. She spoke about the impact on her unit, her staff, institutional effectiveness, morale, and collegiality rather than in overtly personal terms. Helen's leadership role and her location in a well-resourced and prestigious institution informed her experience of and her view of the pandemic.

She reported that four staff members in her unit had become infected with COVID-19, three nurses and a medical assistant. The latter had ongoing symptoms of the disease, or what has been termed "long COVID." She speculated that the infections had occurred outside of clinical settings. Unlike the Johnsons, who struggled with PPE at the beginning of the pandemic, staff in well-resourced, prestigious institutions did not have resource-based problems. In addition to adequate supplies, Helen's employer made amenities available, from isolation rooms for workers who reported COVID symptoms to financial compensation for staff who could not work after exposure or infection. As a leader, Helen organized Zoom "wellness" workshops, where invited speakers discussed coping strategies to deal with stress for employees. In the world described by Helen, nurses faced increased pressure, stress, and strain as the pandemic lingered, but their institution protected and supported them.

A Nigerian nurse who occupied a senior position like Helen's in a HIV/AIDS clinic attached to a different prestigious teaching and research hospital made a similar report. Temi's work also was largely administrative and supervisory, and like Helen, she recalled overwork in the early days of the pandemic as she had to take on more clinical duties due to staff shortages. Her institution also had curtailed the services they offered in their outpatient clinics and had let some staff go. She described feeling like "she was doing the work of ten people at once." Temi also recognized how prepared and advantaged her institution was in comparison to the experiences of her colleagues in state, county, and public hospitals who had to reuse masks and other PPE at the onset of the pandemic. These insights point to the reality of a fragmented health care system and one that is increasingly bifurcated among socioeconomic lines.

There were some things Temi's institution could not protect her from. She recalled fear, particularly at the beginning of the pandemic. She relied on prayer as a coping strategy. Two other nurses described similar fears and using prayer as a coping tool. Miriam spoke about having in-person "get togethers" with a close-knit and trusted group of female friends who supported each other in the later stages of the pandemic. These accounts suggest that, in addition to public health and biomedical approaches to disease prevention, professional workers in health and long-term care also relied on additional "non-scientific" preventive measures and coping strategies such as prayer and informal group therapy.

Temi also described the experiences of colleagues who had become infected with COVID-19, including one colleague who, many months after the initial infection, still suffered from vision and cognitive problems. Describing the toll on African immigrant colleagues who worked in institutions other than her own, Temi explained that many felt they had been abandoned by their institutions and left to battle the disease on their own. Like Helen, Temi believed the pandemic had created unanticipated opportunities. She identified job creation in contract tracing, case management, and more clinical opportunities as the pandemic wore on well into 2021.

The crisis had taken a significant toll on the mental and physical health of nurses as the pandemic persisted. Helen reported that many of her staff experienced burnout. Some, she said, had quit their jobs due to difficulties navigating their work and balancing the care (including home schooling) of their own children during the various phases of the pandemic. While the news media had reported on the stress and burnout faced by health care workers at the "frontlines" of the pandemic (Prasad et al. 2021; Lagasse 2020; Jacobs 2021; Talaee et al. 2020), lesser attention has been paid to the toll on other skilled care workers involved in non-COVID care. Even less is known about how care workers navigated the care of their own family members during the pandemic. In what ways did the pressure, emotional stress, and burnout from COVID-19 result in nurses leaving the profession, and how would these exits related to COVID-19 exacerbate the already chronic shortages of nurses in many parts of the country? (American Association of Colleges of Nursing 2020; Williams 2021). A 2021 *Wall Street Journal* article reported a growing decline in the numbers of paraprofessional nursing home staff during the COVID-19 crisis, with little sign of a coming rebound (Weber 2021). On the other hand, other media reports highlighted the exodus of current nurses because of pandemic-related burnout but also traced a rise in applications to nursing schools inspired, in part, by young people who saw the public health crisis as a challenge and an opportunity (Eaton-Robb 2021; Kowarski 2020). As of the time of the book's writing, I anticipate that health economists, sociologists, nursing, care work, and other scholars are working to piece out the full empirical picture relating to the net gain of new nursing recruits and the net loss of the exodus of current nurses during the pandemic. The net impact on the profession from the loss of long-serving nurses and nurse instructors who take their expertise and many years of experience with them also would be an important topic for ethnographers and other qualitative scholars to bring to light in the years ahead.

All the West African nurses I knew remained in the profession at the time of this book's publication. A few experienced the stressors of being at the "frontlines "of the pandemic, the pressures of witnessing deaths, and feelings of being overwhelmed as cases surged. Some had been infected themselves. A male Sierra Leonean nurse whom I call Sam gained significant attention on Facebook among

Sierra Leoneans in the diaspora in the early days of the pandemic as he discussed his experience after contracting COVID-19. At that time, when the world, including the medical establishment, was unclear about all the symptoms and therapeutics to combat the disease, Sam alerted other Sierra Leonean nurses and care workers about the reality of the threat of COVID-19 and the severity of symptoms. When I contacted him more than a year later, he described the harrowing symptoms he had experienced and spoke of his recovery as a rebirth. "By God's grace I came back to life," he said. He had been exposed in the New York City hospital where he worked as an emergency room/critical care nurse. He described shortages in PPE and critical care equipment, like ventilators. He recalled overflowing emergency rooms with patients lining hallways in March, April, and May 2020, when New York was the epicenter of the virus. He recalled a single night when twenty-two patients in a thirty-bed acute care unit died of the virus.

A year later, in the summer of 2021, Sam had a very different experience of the pandemic. He had taken a leave of absence from his permanent job in New York and was working as a "travel nurse" in response to the chronic shortages that institutions across the nation were facing. In this role, he worked on six- to ten-week rotations in various institutions that needed temporary workers to combat surges in COVID cases. He rationalized his choice to leave his permanent job by saying, "I gotta go make that money." The fact that he was making five times his regular weekly salary as a travel nurse may explain why Sam thought the pandemic had been "a curse and a blessing."

I spoke to or became aware of other African nurses also working as travel nurses. One of these nurses reported through social media that she and some colleagues left their jobs in Georgia to work for a period of 140 days in an intensive care unit in Texas at a time of a peak in COVID infections. Unlike nurses like Sam, who quit their jobs permanently and of their own volition, this nurse's relocation appeared to be initiated by her employer to help embattled institutions in other parts of the country. Another nurse quit her job in New Jersey and signed up as a travel nurse in California. Like Sam, she cited higher wages as the cause of her decision. In a matter-of-fact tone, she told me about walking away from her job to seek financial rewards. In this case, as was the case for Sam, the financial rewards in working in temporary placements as a travel nurse outweighed the costs of living temporarily in another state away from family and working as temporary staff in care related to COVID-19.

As we move past the emergency response stage of the pandemic, and as the focus moves from mitigating the outbreaks of COVID-19 and its variants to a potential future in which the virus is endemic in populations, it will be worthwhile to provide detailed analysis that tracks the full temporal context and scale of the virus. A post-mortem analysis that accounts for the impact of the various waves of the virus on different groups of workers will be particularly germane.

Which workers bore the brunt of intensive COVID-19 care, and in which periods were the stresses most intense? Which groups of workers were able to opt out of the profession, and what informed their choices? In what ways did racial disparities play out? What were the intersections of race, class, gender, ethnicity, and immigration status in the experience of the pandemic? Which groups of nurses and other frontline care workers were able to capitalize on structural needs and demands, and in what ways did the pandemic provide unanticipated opportunities and consequences? Did the uncomfortable divides between "real nurses" versus "opportunists" discussed in chapter 5 play out in the pandemic? Were some nurses committed to the care of critically ill and dying, and did some see within COVID-19 an opportunity to "make money?" These are uncomfortable questions, and I hope reality will not reflect such stark divides.

We do know that the surge in COVID-19 cases in various geographies exacerbated existing staff shortages and placed current nurses under strain. These shortages created a demand for temporary workers and a concomitant raise in wages to attract workers. Some of the nurses I interviewed or got to know met this demand and were better off financially for it. They also hinted at a chilly reception by the staff nurses in the institutions where they worked temporarily. A fuller account that takes seriously the interpersonal dynamics at play between these well-paid travel nurses and the nurses who stayed in their jobs to combat the pandemic while receiving their existing pay levels is needed. An analysis that investigates the tensions, strains, and potential points of solidarity between these two groups of workers thrown together in the COVID crisis will be particularly useful, as will be policy-oriented research directed toward building a robust and resilient nursing staff to take care of everyday health care needs as well as to combat future pandemics. Examining the impact on immigrant-owned and other businesses that cater to a low-income, marginalized, largely racial minority populations also would be an important ethnographic arena for researchers to follow.

COVID-19 plunged the U.S. health care system and, indeed, the entire society into crisis. As workers in institutional and private health care settings, the subjects of my book who, in a lot of ways, were "unintentional" care workers, became direct players in the tragedy that unfolded. Some combatted the virus as business owners and leaders or as administrators in prestigious institutions. Many others were foot soldiers in hospitals, nursing homes, and private homes. Their experiences were shaped by the context within which they worked and the roles they occupied. In these pages, I have laid out some of the preliminary themes that characterize their experiences. I also have raised some questions that future research agendas interested in the health and long-term care work force in general would do well to explore. For scholars, policymakers, and the general population alike, we might find in the catastrophes endured and the lessons learned during the COVID-19 crisis some of the tools we need to work toward creating a more caring society.

APPENDIX A
Methodological Appendix

I collected data for this study by using three primary methods: interviews, participant observation at the business I call Worldwide, and field observations at seven other West African-owned home care agencies. I chose the Washington, DC, metropolitan area as a site for this study because African immigrants are concentrated in this area. In 2019, the Washington, DC, metropolitan area was second only to the greater New York City area as the metro areas with the largest number of Sub-Saharan African immigrants (Lorenzi and Batalova 2022). Besides the significant concentrations of Sub-Saharan Africans in the DC area compared to others, the presence of West African churches, restaurants, grocery and food stores, and other businesses and organizations illustrate a vibrant and growing ethnic community. These ethnic community organizations and institutions were useful to gain access to this population and as a prism through which to understand their social worlds.

DATA COLLECTION

I collected data during the summer months, May through August, from 2010 to 2012, with a different focus in each period. In summer 2015, I returned to the field and conducted more participant observation and interviews.

The first two phases (summer 2010 and 2011) were centered around in-depth interviews conducted with female registered and licensed practical nurses I met at churches attended by different national groups within the West African community. These churches were sites of recruitment. I also used personal and social networks and professional organizations in the area to recruit nurse participants.

In summer 2012, I turned my attention to the businesses that West African immigrants had established. I chose home care and disability support businesses that were owned and operated by West Africans as work sites to conduct field observation, rather than other institutional settings like hospitals or nursing homes, to systematically map out and trace the processes that have facilitated the clustering of West Africans in health care and to investigate their dual role as laborers, entrepreneurs, and labor brokers responsible for channeling coethnics into health care work. In this phase (summer 2012), I was an "intermittent observer" (Purser 2009) at most of these worksites. I visited on paydays, when workers congregated to receive paychecks, and frequented the offices during normal business hours, introducing myself and my research to both care workers and administrative staff. During these visits, I observed the goings-on in the offices, including the interactions between the staff and individuals who visited to inquire about job openings or submitted job applications. I interviewed some owners, administrators, and managers of these businesses. I also recruited male and female care workers I met causally in waiting rooms, elevators, etc., and more formally at job trainings. My usual approach was to briefly introduce myself and my research to potential participants. If they were willing and interested, I gave them my university's Institutional Review Board-approved information sheet explaining my study and took their contact information. I then followed up with a phone call to schedule more formal interviews. In a few cases, I conducted interviews on the spot after gaining informed consent.[1]

In this phase, I started participant observation at Worldwide. To immerse myself in the setting and to understand the business of health care provision, I volunteered my services as an unpaid intern and assisted with clerical and administrative tasks. I spent time at the day program, where I observed the care provided by the staff, who were mainly Sierra Leonean. I also attended training and orientation sessions for new health care paraprofessional staff and accompanied senior administrative staff to meetings with local government officers and other actors in the Washington, DC, health care services bureaucracy.

The final phase was summer 2015, when I returned to Worldwide and continued the activities just outlined. I also interviewed more of their staff. It was in this final phase that I conducted most of the interviews with DSPs. Focusing on Worldwide, a Sierra Leonean-owned company, led to an oversampling of Sierra Leonean interview participants.

ACCESSING AND STUDYING IMMIGRANT POPULATIONS

To gain access to this population and to conduct field research, I used multiple entry points. I recruited most of the nurse participants at three evangelical churches that cater to distinct West African populations. All churches were in Maryland. One church had a Nigerian pastor and a predominantly Nigerian congregation, though other West African nationals as well as nationals from other countries were represented. A second church was a predominantly Ghanaian congregation headed by a Ghanaian pastor. I recruited participants in a third church with a predominantly Liberian congregation and leadership. Many members of the congregation in the identified churches worked as nurses and health care support staff. The nurses worked in different types of institutions: hospitals, nursing homes, physicians' offices, and as visiting home nurses.

The decision to use churches as an entry point into the community was a practical one, as many members of the targeted population attended church on a regular basis. The church also served as the center of their social worlds. For instance, in addition to Sunday church services, there were weekday prayer meetings and bible studies as well as social events, such as church picnics. Attending these events in the beginning of my field work gave me some insights into the strength of their communities and informal social networks. I also approached church leaders, such as pastors and respected women leaders, "ethnic brokers," or conduits into this community who identified participants in their congregations who fit my selection criteria. Going through church elders allowed me gain the trust of potential participants who might not otherwise be inclined to discuss matters such as immigration status with strangers.

While the church granted me access to the community and a convenient site to recruit nurse participants for the study, I note some methodological limitations that stem from the possible selection bias of the group. Given that I used evangelical churches as sites to recruit participants, I tended to oversample people who were evangelical or "born-again" Christians with a particular world view and religious approach. This fact may have influenced their views, especially as it relates to their subjective understandings of work. To mitigate this potential selection bias, I extended my points of entry to include drawing from my personal networks, tapping into ethnic organizations in the area, and using African-owned home care and disability support agencies to reach other care workers beside Christian nurses, and to understand the varied spheres of life of this group.

I conducted field research at home care and disability support agencies (seven offices) and recruited a few nurses, but mostly qualified disability support professionals, at these offices. The agencies were located predominantly in Washington, DC, and catered to DC residents. In these agencies, I acted as an "intermittent" rather than participant observer. I became aware of these agencies early in my research through the interviews I conducted with nurses. I found that several West African women nurses also worked as visiting home nurses. Sometimes, in addition to their regular job at a hospital or nursing home, they would pick up shifts and "hours" through home care or nurse staffing agencies embedded in their ethnic networks.

Drawing from a list of home care agencies obtained from the Washington, DC, Department of Health website, I found that about half of the administrators listed as contact persons had what I read as African sounding last names. Using that initial list, I started visiting the agencies listed, where I started informal conversations with the staff.[2] I also observed the happenings in the offices. A few agencies were more receptive to my visits than others, and I limited my later visits to those. I made sure to drop by on paydays and in-service training sessions, where I got the opportunity to meet and interact with the staff—nurses as well as home health aides. I also conducted formal interviews with administrators, such as the directors of nursing, program administrators, and general managers of those agencies. I also attended a few in-service training sessions for three agencies that granted me access. Through this, I was able to observe the types of training and disciplining that some of these institutions seek to impart on their workers; in this case, their predominantly African staff.

I concentrated my efforts at Worldwide (the day program) as a site where I had repeated access to their staff. I developed a strong rapport with the administrators there, perhaps because they were second-generation immigrants socialized largely in American educational and social institutions and thus understood that my project would shed intellectual light on the contributions of West Africans to U.S. health care. We also connected due to our shared identities as Black women with immigrant backgrounds living in America. One of the administrators told me that they were invested in supporting another Sierra Leonean woman who was earning a PhD. Unlike the other agencies, they gave me the most unrestricted access to interview their staff as well as to conduct continued participant observation.

Finally, I tapped into formal (community organizations and professional associations) and informal (family and friends) networks to recruit participants for this study. I identified a few women from existing family networks but also from contacts made during previous visits to the Washington, DC, area. Using snowball sampling methods, I asked these initial contacts to identity co-workers, friends, and relatives to be added to the study. Family and national gatherings, country independence celebrations, picnics, birthdays, and graduation celebrations all were social events that became opportunities for data collection. I found that these celebrations, at which a sizeable proportion of the attendees happened to be nurses or other care workers, provided me with a place where I could recruit participants and observe the interactions among people within the African community. Being invited to these social events and others, such as special church services, was an extension of community spirit, welcome, solidarity, and a sign I had developed good rapport. Finally, the African Women's Cancer Awareness Association (AWCAA) and the African Immigrant and Refugee Foundation (AIRF) are two organizations whose programming and work I became familiar with. The programs and services offered by these two organizations provided yet another way for me to gain more access to the communities and to gain their trust.

INTERVIEWS

I conducted semi-structured, in-depth qualitative interviews with sixty-three first-generation immigrants from Sierra Leone, Nigeria, Ghana, Cameroon, and

Liberia. I also interviewed three second-generation Sierra Leonean and Nigerian immigrants. Interviewees all lived and worked in the Washington, DC, metropolitan area. They worked within various occupational settings in the health and long-term care industries (hospitals, nursing homes, group homes, day program centers, and private homes), and cared for a diverse group of care recipients. Fifty-four interview subjects were women and twelve were men. Interviewees ranged in age from early twenties to late sixties. I interviewed two nurse practitioners, two nursing administrators, twenty-five registered nurses, twelve licensed practical nurses, four certified nursing assistants, eleven qualified intellectual disability support professionals/house managers of residential care homes, and ten administrators/owners of nurse staffing and recruitment agencies. The sample is representative of national-level data that has shown the health care industry as one of the niche areas in the service industry in which African immigrants are concentrated. This data also shows that Africans are represented in professional and paraprofessional sectors of the industry. For instance, a 2012 study noted that African men and women workers were more likely to report holding jobs as health care practitioners and in other health care support occupations. Indeed, "compared to male immigrants overall, African-born male workers were more likely to report working as health care practitioners and in other health care support occupations" (McCabe 2012). At present, though a small share of the total immigrant population (4.5 percent), Africans make up 12 percent of the immigrant share of the healthcare labor force (Batalova 2020; Echevarria-Estrada and Batalova 2019). Within health care occupations, African immigrants are more likely to work as registered nurses, and in health care support occupations such as home health aides, certified nursing assistants, and disability support professionals (Batalova 2020).

The nurses I interviewed had a mixture of degrees and educational qualifications; some even had multiple qualifications they had earned after migration. The majority had bachelor's of science degrees (BSNs), but a few had associate's degrees. Five had master's of science in nursing (MSNs) and two were nurse practitioners (NPs). A couple had master's degrees in business administration (MBA) in addition to their registered nurse qualifications, and one in my sample had a master's in public administration (MPA). A few had a combination of degrees; for example, one RN was also BSN/MBA. Nine of forty-one professional nurses were trained and qualified nurses in their home countries. They had to go through retraining and credentialing procedures that necessitated further education upon migration. All nurses also had to pass a national licensing examination to obtain a nursing license. The disability support professionals had a mixture of pre- and post-migration qualifications but were less likely than the nurses to have furthered their education in the United States. Most in the sample (nurses and DSPS) who migrated as adults had at least a bachelor's degree prior to migration. A few had earned bachelor's degrees in the United States or, in one case, in England, before migrating to the United States. One QIDP had earned a master's in public health degree (MPH) after migration.

Prior to migration, study participants who migrated as adults held middle-class jobs as teachers, accountants, business owners, engineers, etc. and occupied several administrative positions. The high educational attainment and human capital of the group sampled for this study is representative of national statistics that have reported that African immigrants as a group possess the highest levels of educational attainment of all immigrant groups to the United States (Batalova 2020; McCabe 2012; Arthur 2009). Despite these premigration educational qualifications, in addition to starting their careers in the bottom ranks of the health care industry in the United States, some reported having done other low-wage service work in the United States (e.g., office cleaning, taxi driving, serving in fast-food restaurants, petty trading, babysitting, and domestic work) before entering the health care industry.

At the time of the interviews, all respondents who agreed to speak on the matter reported legal immigration status. Study participants had lived in the United States for varying amounts of time. The most recently arrived had lived in the United States for only one year, while the participant with the longest tenure had lived in the United States for forty years. The average length of time all study participants had lived in the United States was seventeen years. Eight people in the sample had migrated before the age of twelve, forming part of what has been termed the "1.5 generation." An additional twelve had migrated as young adults immediately after they completed high school. Most of the participants who migrated in childhood or early adulthood reported middle-class backgrounds in their home countries.

The care worker interviews were informed by an interview guide that asked open-ended questions about motivations and experiences of migration; work histories; pathways into and experiences in care work; relations with clients, co-workers, and supervisors; job satisfaction and difficulties; and future job prospects. For the female participants, I conducted interviews in their homes or at churches, the group homes and offices operated by Worldwide, offices of other agencies, and immigrant social gatherings. All the interviews with male participants occurred at the day program run by Worldwide; at the offices of other home care or disability support businesses; or, in a few cases, the residential homes where they cared for groups of individuals. I followed a similar procedure for my interviews with administrators of the home care and disability support businesses. In those interviews, the interview guide consisted of open-ended questions regarding background and education in health care and/or health care administration, qualifications in the field, and descriptions of daily work experiences. I also asked questions relating to their clients' demographics; funding; training, disciplining, and recruitment of nursing and home health care and disability support staff; the ethnic and national makeup of staff; and their assessments of African nurses and DSPs. These in-depth interviews with health care industry administrators were important for discovering how industry actors conceptualized their work and their relationships with clientele (coethnics and other staff, clients/care recipients), relevant organizations, institutions, and actors such as DC and federal government agencies, Medicaid and Medicare, and private insurance companies.

DATA ANALYSIS

I started my data analysis almost as soon as I started interviews. Even though I recorded interviews, I also took detailed notes during each interview. For example, I jotted down details about respondents' hometown, educational background, intriguing work experiences and interactions, and poignant phrases or expressions that stood out to me. After each interview, I revisited these notes and then typed up a one-paragraph summary of the subject's background, any information that stood out in their history and biography, preliminary themes that came up in the interview, any observations that were poignant, or any questions that emerged from my handwritten notes. I quickly began noticing repetition in the themes, which then provided me with ideas on which to build and develop as I continued further interviews. I also used further interviews to clarify questions that were emerging in my notes. These paragraph summaries were useful in letting me know when I was approaching the point of data saturation, even before I had started the formal process of transcribing, coding, and analyzing the data.

Conducting the interviews in phases helped with data analysis as I transcribed the interviews after each round of data collection, ensuring that the data was always manageable. My handwritten notes and typed paragraph summaries helped evoke vivid memories of the people I had met, even as my time in the field became more distant. I frequently revisited transcripts of interviews as well as my contemporaneous notes, ensuring an intimacy with the data that continued well into the writing phase of the project.

I read over each transcript and systematically analyzed the data, line by line, using open coding (Emerson, Fretz, and Shaw 2011; Lofland et al. 2006). This process led me to generate over 200 codes, which were further defined into subcodes. Examples of codes with associated subcodes (italicized and in parenthesis) are: role of social networks (*social networks and info about health care; social networks in sparking interest; social networks in job placement; networks of women going into care together*); positives of the job; (*positives—financial rewards; positives—flexibility; positives—means to an end; positives—many opportunities in nursing; positives—job fulfillment*); affect/emotion in care work (*compassion versus rationality; compassion—ethic of care; humanity/humanity of condition/empathy*); family discourses in care (*treating care receivers as family; saying employers are like family; work versus family discourse; saying it's work not family*). I also highlighted sections of coded text containing quotes that I believed illuminated subsequent themes particularly well. I then typed up the codes and subcodes into Microsoft Excel with accompanying page numbers of transcripts where they appeared and respondent initials, helping me match the codes with the interview transcripts. This process also generated a tally of the most recurring codes and subcodes. These were later sorted into chapters through focused coding (Loftland et al. 2006). I used a grounded theory approach to data collection, which allowed categories and themes to emerge from the data, while maintaining connections to the existing literature to draw theoretical conclusions (Strauss and Corbin 1994).

PARTICIPANT OBSERVATION

In contrast to my field observations at other agencies, where my activities were limited to a few in-service staff trainings, conducting interviews with the administrators and managers, and recruiting care worker participants, I formed a more concrete idea of the actual social organization of health care work through participant observation at Worldwide Services, Inc. I describe this business and detail some of my observations in chapters 3 and 4.

My experience with Worldwide began when I introduced myself and my research to Miriam, the director of nursing, and suggested I would volunteer my services in exchange for permission to "hang around and observe [their] activities as well as to interview staff." Miriam enthusiastically agreed, and she suggested I work as an unpaid "intern." She asked that I obtain a DSP certification, a process that entailed completing the online training and certification organized by the DC Department of Disability Services and undergo a criminal background check. With certification in hand, I was then permitted to sit in on staff meetings and other meetings, such as the individualized support planning meetings, where I was privy to some confidential client matters.

I spent on average three days a week at the day program, from around 9:30 A.M. to 4 P.M. for three months in summer 2012 and two and a half months in summer 2015. (I visited other agencies on the remaining two days of the week). I interacted with the predominantly Sierra Leonean staff that consisted of counselors, DSPs, case managers, QIDPs, and, on a few occasions, the Sierra Leonean medical doctor in charge of care. I also met some of the house managers who came into the office on occasion. I shadowed the on-site nurse as she gave medications. I gained access to the classroom settings for the clients and observed staff interactions with the clients. I also sat in on staff nurse meetings and training sessions. I attended annual plan of care meetings, meetings that brought together a team of caregivers and other stakeholders responsible for the well-being of patients, many of whom were wards of the state. I sat on the sidelines with many other staff members while the QIDP, RN, medical doctor, legal representative of the individual, etc. discussed the case and created a plan of care for the individual. In addition to the information learned in the formal proceedings, I had informal chats with staff members not participating in the discussion. I learned a lot from those interactions; for instance, staff clarified what certain acronyms meant or gave me some context for understanding unfolding events. I also attended industry meetings with the administrators at Worldwide (with local DC authorities or other care administrators). Like the plan of care meetings, while I did not speak or formally participate in these meetings, I would have appeared to onlookers as part of the team at Worldwide. At the meetings at Worldwide, I did not stand out from staff, since many of the QIDPs and managerial staff wore plain clothes and not scrubs, or jeans and T-shirts emblazoned with the Worldwide logo that the counselors wore as uniforms. In these meetings, I always took detailed handwritten notes on what I saw and heard. I jotted down my general observations in a small note pad that I carried around throughout my time at Worldwide. I usually typed up my field notes at the end of each workday. I added reflections on what I had seen and heard in those more detailed notes.

In my voluntary role as intern, I assisted with a few clerical duties. For instance, one task was to create a database of the aides who had been trained as medical technicians; that is, certified to administer medication. To get this information, I had to call the various house managers on the phone, who then provided the names of the aides who met that criterion. I, then, entered the information in a database. I reported directly to Miriam. Apart from tasks such as the one just described, I was given complete autonomy by the agency administrators, and spent most of my time engaged in research-related activities. While I did not personally provide care, and while my role as "intern" was largely limited, I learned a lot about the job by being immersed in the setting. I got a sense of how work was organized at this Sierra Leonean agency that hired a predominantly Sierra Leonean staff. I also got to observe staff interactions with mainstream institutions and actors. Miriam and Malaika, the DON and VP at Worldwide, routinely introduced me to staff members as a graduate student working on a "paper," although I think staff members understood that to mean I was a college student working on a term paper. When I returned in 2015, they introduced me as "Dr. Showers" and told their staff I was writing a book. Many of the Sierra Leoneans expressed pride that one of their own was a "doctor." They appeared happy to consent to interviews to help with my book. Apart from when I approached staff for interviews, I tried to be as unobstructive as possible during my time at Worldwide, and most of the time, I believe my presence went largely unnoticed.

PERSONAL LOCATION AND FINAL REFLECTIONS

Like some of my research participants, I once worked as a home health aide. In my case, I was very bad at it. In summer 2007, I had just completed a master's degree and had been accepted into a PhD program starting in the fall of that year.

I needed a job that would tide me over till my studies and modest graduate stipend commenced. A friend of mine, a daughter of Ghanaian immigrants, told me to become a home health aide. My friend, *a care pioneer*, advised I sign up with a recruitment agency who would then broker my services as a home health aide. Riddled with anxiety, I asked my friend whether I would be a suitable candidate for a home health aide position, and she told me, "Don't worry, they take everybody." And so began my short stint as a home health aide.

I signed up with a recruitment agency in upstate New York. As I recall, the recruitment agency offered a no-cost training, which lasted about two weeks. Most of the training consisted of in-class instruction and then a two-day practicum where we would test our skills working with the residents of a selected nursing home. If we passed written tests and quizzes administered in class, made it through the nursing home portion, and passed a criminal background check, we would be certified as home health aides and we would begin our tenure as paid hourly employees of the agency.

The staff in that agency in upstate New York were mostly white women, and our instructor was an older white woman who was a registered nurse. My fellow trainees were African American and white women. According to my recollection, the class was evenly divided between Black and white women, and there were no men or foreign-born women in my cohort. Aside from vague memories about lessons on meal preparation and nutrition; how to take blood pressure or calculate a pulse; and how to make "hospital corners" on bed sheets, I do not recall much about the specifics of the training or didactic materials we received. (See Schweid 2021 for a scholarly account of home health training and the experiences of home health aides.)

A few general memories of that time, however, will always stay with me. One was that, while I excelled in the written portion of the exams, I struggled with the practical side of things. I recalled one lesson where we were taught how to make a bed with a person (presumably a bedridden patient) still in it. The instructor demonstrated the technique with a dummy, and we were to take turns practicing our skills with our classmates serving as the bedridden patient. The goal was to gently roll the patient to one side, neatly adjust the sheets on the now unoccupied side of the bed, and repeat the process for the other side. I remember the whole class bursting into laughter when it was my turn. My attempts to follow the techniques I had observed ended with me wrapping up my fellow trainee like a mummy. While the rest of the class experienced the whole episode as a big joke, the instructor sharply reprimanded me, saying something about how that would not do in a real-world situation.

Another incident I never will forget occurred at the end of our training when we were asked to work in a nursing home. I was supposed to give one of the nursing home residents a shower. Armed with the theoretical knowledge about how to give a shower (e.g., always start from the cleanest part of the body—that is, the face—

and work to the most unclean part), I helped the care receiver into the shower. Frail, she had to sit on a stool, and I started the shower by holding the hand-held shower nozzle over her body. As soon as the water hit her body, she shrieked. I then realized the water was ice cold. Panicked and horrified, my hands started to shake violently. I then had water all over the bathroom floor. . . . and on my distressed care recipient. The whole episode was, in a word, terrible. Surely, I thought, the agency would send me packing after this. But, on the contrary, I continued my day at the nursing home and received my home health aide certification at the end. My friend was right. They really do "take everybody." I learned from my practical experience, however, that the labor cannot be performed by just anybody.

That summer, I travelled large distances, and I traversed various worlds as a home health aide. I cared for different groups of patients and worked in various conditions and circumstances. For instance, I worked for some patients, mostly African American, who lived in apartments in public housing complexes in the city. Those clients typically received only about two hours of care, and my tasks were typically to prepare meals (breakfast, lunch, or dinner, depending on time of day), help with feeding, or do light housework or laundry. The agency usually pooled these care recipients and their needs, so I tended to work for a few clients within the same housing complex or in neighboring complexes.

A couple of care recipients in this group stand out in my memory. One was an older African American woman, a diabetic, whose legs recently had been amputated due to complications of the disease. She was experiencing "phantom limb pain." I remember one conversation where she told me she could feel every single one of her toes, despite the missing limb. I still remember her visceral reaction and the pain etched on her face. Another client and situation that stood out to me involved a middle-aged African American man who I recall as able-bodied. I don't recall the specifics of his diagnoses or medical conditions. My tasks were to do laundry and light housework. I usually entered the apartment and carried my duties undisturbed as he remained in the living room playing with his extensive toy train collection.

I also cared for white clients in working-class neighborhoods, and others in more affluent neighborhoods. The latter often were the care receivers who could afford overnight care or pay for many hours of care during the day. Sometimes, they had round-the-clock care, and home health aides would rotate twelve-hour shifts. When I worked overnight shifts, I would arrive in time to help a family member put the care recipient to bed. I would spend the night on a couch in the living room or in a spare bedroom. I don't recall any dramatic incidents over the night, but I did observe a certain set of relationships with this clientele that reflect the intersections of race, class, gender, nationality, and global inequality that I have engaged in this book.

I worked with a family in which the care recipient was an older man. Shortly after I started work, he was referred to hospice care. I sat quietly as his wife and adult daughters discussed the financial burdens of his care with a representative of the hospice facility. Later that day, I watched as he was taken away from his home, the home he had shared with his partner for decades, presumably for the last time. Distraught, his wife hugged and tearfully kissed him as he was carried away. I sat silently observing this family go through what was probably one of the worst days of their life, all the while seemingly invisible.

As I reflected on these experiences later, and while writing this book, I am struck that my experiences exemplify many of the established themes of servitude and invisibility in domestic work. Judith Rollins' (1987) classic on Black women domestics and their white employers explored the general invisibility that Black women experienced as they worked in the homes of their white employers. Like my experience described above, these women were privy to the most intimate of family circumstances while being simultaneously overlooked and ignored. Other scholars, as I have shown in this book, have explored the themes of servitude in elder care and home care. Regarding servitude, I remember a case where an older white woman care recipient followed me around as I vacuumed her living room, pointing out spots I had supposedly missed. She mentioned I was lucky she had taken the trouble to point out my errors rather than report me to the agency. I still remember the feeling of humiliation and anger I felt, emotions that have been explored at length in Cati Coe's ethnography on African immigrant elder care workers.

The complications and contradictions of class, race, and gender identities in care were evident in one final interaction I will share here. I worked in the home of an older Jewish woman, and a couple of times I encountered her adult son. One day, I was sitting in the living room when the family started going through old family photos displayed on a side table. The son pointed out old black-and-white pictures of his late dad and his brother. Just trying to make polite conversation, I pointed out a particular photo of the son (as a young man) with the late Israeli prime minister Golda Meir, asking about the story behind the photo. They were visibly stunned that the home health aide had recognized and named a potentially obscure political figure. I told them that I was, in fact, a graduate student at a well-regarded local university. From then on, there was a noticeable difference in how the family treated me. I spent most of the remainder of my time with the mother watching the news, and I recall that most of our conversations centered around the news of the day and political matters.

My relationship with care work is, therefore, intensely personal as well as intellectual. As a Black, African, immigrant woman in the United States, I have experiential similarities with many of my research participants. I share a nationality and some ethnic similarity with the Sierra Leonean participants. I have a Nigerian (Yoruba) first name, which made for a unique point of connection with the Nigerians, many of whom were ethnic Yorubas. Hailing from the same continent with the Ghanaians and Cameroonians, and a country that shared a border with the Liberians, made for good small talk with the rest of the participants and helped lighten the mood before we dove into the interviews. I share, therefore, what feminist scholars have called an "insider status" with my research participants, or what sociologist Sheba George (2005) has called "autobiographical proximity" to the research. This "insider" status helped with my access to and relationship with the research population (Collins 1991; Devault 1999).

Having worked as a home health aide, albeit briefly, also aided in gaining rapport and facilitated comfortable relationships with many of my research participants. A few times during the interviews, respondents visibly relaxed when I shared that I had worked as a home health aide. I could see this helped ease some of the discomfort they felt in discussing their early experiences with direct care work. Knowledge of basic medical technology and terminology also helped the interview process. I recall one incident when a nurse mentioned a Hoyer lift[3] and I nodded in agreement because we had received basic instruction about its use in my home health aide class. These moments of understanding and recognition helped ease the relational aspects of conducting this research. These brief moments of understanding notwithstanding, I do not want to overstate my similarities with my research subjects. Performing paid care work for one summer, a position I abandoned rather unceremoniously to start my studies in a doctoral program, is very different from the circumstances of the individuals in this research. They were compelled to enter care work because of displacement in the U.S. labor market due to the erasure of their human capital. For them, care work was not just a temporary "occupational detour" on their way to their real careers. As I have shown in the book, direct care work was, for many, simply the "least bad" of many bad employment options they had undertaken after migration.

When I set out to conduct this research, my goal was to focus on West African women direct care workers. However, I found that, through my interactions in the churches detailed earlier in this section, I was steered by "ethnic gatekeepers," the pastors and leaders of the church, to middle-class nurses, whom they believed were better representatives of the community. I also noted that some of the immigrants who were current direct care workers actively avoided me or refused my attempts to reach out regarding this research. I can only surmise that some were wary due to their possible undocumented immigration status. Direct care workers also worked extremely long hours and probably had even less time to spare for interviews than their professional counterparts. Had I centered my empirical attention on current direct care workers rather than the professional workers who had previously worked as direct care workers, the experiences I would have shared in this book would have been closer to the one I myself experienced as a home health aide. Rather, the story I have told is one of initial labor displacement after migration; pain, humiliation, and class ambivalence after incorporation in direct care work; and entry into professional health care and accompanying professional success that most of the individuals encountered.

While my insider status granted me many advantages, as I have noted, this position also complicated my relationships with the research participants. As an insider, I believe some participants were hesitant to share details about their family life, finances, and parenting troubles. While many scholars have found their insider position an advantage, as participants feel comfortable talking to someone who truly understands their experiences (see Banerjee 2022 for a discussion on this in relation to immigrant identities), in my case, I felt that being part of the West African (Sierra Leonean) immigrant community meant that people were wary of divulging intimate details of their personal or family lives or "telling their business" to someone who could potentially judge them or, worse, gossip about them. While I stressed the standards of confidentiality to which I was bound as a researcher, participants were forthcoming with their professional lives but did not provide many details about their marriages (especially when contracted to legalize their status) or their earnings, as well as their family lives.

I found out later through my interactions in the churches and other community institutions that discussing immigration with coethnics was difficult. Divulging one's immigration status was rarely done, as community members believed that one's undocumented status could become the basis of threats of being turned over to the authorities by family members and domestic partners and make one vulnerable to exploitation. While all research subjects who agreed to interviews were legally authorized immigrants at the time of our interactions, my insider status did not mean that participants always were willing to trust me with the specifics of how they had navigated the immigration process. In those cases where interviewees communicated that they felt uncomfortable discussing how they had navigated their move from temporary, non-immigrant status to permanent residency or naturalized citizenship status, I was respectful of their concerns and stopped that line of questioning. Also, their discussions of problems encountered at work in mainstream institutions focused on the racial and ethnic discrimination they encountered, but there were surprisingly few accounts of sexual harassment and sexism at work. Participants' accounts of their experiences as employees in ethnic-owned businesses also were strikingly positive. No one discussed exploitation, mistreatment by employers, or misgivings about their work in those settings. The latter points could mean that this truly was their experience, but I have pondered the possibility that there was a limit to the level of trust I had developed with my subjects as a researcher. I acknowledge this as a possible limitation of the data I have reported.

Considering my "insider status" led me also to interrogate my gender identity. I realized I had more ease with the women participants in the study. I had no concerns or misgivings when it came to visiting their homes, and I even conducted interviews in the late evening or at night in my attempts to work around their schedules. However, with the male participants, all the interviews were conducted in their workplaces and, in one case, at a restaurant where the research participant and I met for a late lunch. While I found I developed a rapport with the men, I also remembered that in at least a couple of instances I was subject to inappropriate comments that I found deeply uncomfortable. I believe that the fact that I was African myself allowed for professional boundaries to be crossed in a way that may not have been the case if I were native-born American.

As I conclude this book, I have tried to reflect on my relative privilege as someone who had received a U.S. college education and was upwardly mobile as a graduate student and, later, a tenure-track assistant professor when I conducted the research. My class location in the United States, as well as my middle-class upbringing in Sierra Leone, also influenced my interactions with my research participants and the story I have told in this book. This relative privilege put me in an "insider-outsider" position vis a vis my research participants (Beoku-Betts 1994). I was able to relate to many of my immigrant research participants, but I felt most comfortable with those who were of the 1.5 generation or, like me, had migrated as young adults. As I have discussed earlier, I was able to form the most comfortable working relationship with the second-generation children of the business owners at Worldwide because of our shared identities as middle-class, professional, Black, African women who had benefitted from an American undergraduate and graduate education. Their warmth, camaraderie, and support for this research helped me unpack the role of African immigrants as health care entrepreneurs, and their generosity in providing access to their staff greatly enriched the data I was able to gather on the disability professionals. The result is the story I have told here: a focus on how middle-class West African immigrants are produced, repackaged, and deployed as health care workers after migration.

APPENDIX B
Types of Health Care Jobs

NURSING

- Nurse practitioners (NP): professionals who work in clinics, nursing homes, hospitals, or private offices. They provide a wide range of primary and preventive health care services, prescribe medications, and diagnose and treat common minor illnesses and injuries. Generally, NPs must hold a master's degree or higher and pass appropriate certification examinations.
- Registered nurses (RN): work in clinics, nursing homes, hospitals, and in private homes. In addition to providing direct patient care, such as performing physical exams and health histories, administering medications, providing wound care, etc., they provide health promotion, counseling, and education. They coordinate care in collaboration with a wide array of health care professionals. They direct and supervise the care delivered by nursing personnel with lesser credentials. In all states and the District of Columbia, RNs must graduate from an approved registered nurse program and pass a national licensing examination. Maryland requires annual license renewal, and the District of Columbia requires it biannually.
- Licensed practical nurses (LPN), also known as licensed vocational nurses (LVNs) in California and Texas: complement the health care team by providing basic and routine care consistent with their education under the direction of an RN or an advanced practicing nurse, such as an NP. Most LPNs provide basic bedside care. They take vital signs such as temperature, blood pressure, pulse, and respiration. They also treat bedsores, prepare and give injections and enemas, apply dressings, monitor catheters, and perform other routine health care treatments. All states and the District of Columbia require that LPNs pass a licensing examination after completing a state-approved practical nursing program. The practical nursing program usually takes one year. The frequency of license renewal is the same in the District of Columbia in Maryland as for RNs.

- Certified nursing assistants (CNA) and home health aides (HHA): both are paraprofessionals; the main difference is that the former work in institutional settings and the latter in home settings. They also are known as nursing aides, geriatric aides, unlicensed assistive personnel, or hospital attendants. CNAs and HHAs perform routine tasks under the supervision of nursing and medical personnel. They answer patients' call lights or signals to ascertain patients' needs. They perform the activities of daily living (ADL), which include bathing, dressing, brushing hair, brushing teeth, serving meals, assisting patients with eating, etc. In some states, CNAs and HHAs can perform routine health care tasks under the direction of other health care professionals. In many cases, nursing homes and other health care institutions hire CNAs with no qualifications on the condition that they complete a minimum of seventy-five hours of mandatory training and pass a competency evaluation program within four months of employment. Aides who complete the program are certified and placed on the state registry of nursing aides.

DISABILITY SUPPORT

- Disability Support Professionals (DSP): provide hands-on care, such as feeding and bathing, and help with mobility for adults with physical and intellectual disabilities.
- Qualified Intellectual Disability Professionals (QIDP): responsible for integrating, coordinating, and monitoring each client's active treatment. They are staff who possess at least one year of experience working directly with persons with intellectual disabilities or other developmental disabilities.

ACKNOWLEDGMENTS

Writing this book has been a remarkable intellectual, emotional, and personal journey that has expanded over a long stretch of time and space. Throughout, a network of people stood with me. I would like to thank those who have helped launch this journey and accompanied me along the way.

I am deeply indebted to my research participants, without whom this work would not have been possible. Even though I cannot reference them by name, I am grateful to each one of them. I cherish the sacrifice of their time as well as the warmth with which they invited me into their homes or places of work and shared deeply personal stories and experiences. I hope they can find within these pages a true representation of their experiences, struggles, and successes.

I would like to thank my mentors and advisers who inspired my intellectual curiosity and guided me toward the questions and concerns of this book. I am particularly grateful to Linda Carty, who gave me the language to put my own history of migration, as well as my broader questions and ideas, into intellectual context, thus setting me on the path that would result in this book. I will forever be grateful for her acumen, activism, kindness, and care. Without Linda's unwavering support, this book would not have been possible. I also am grateful to Marjorie Devault, who always believed in this project. It was in her qualitative methods course that I began to hatch the plans for data collection. I always enjoyed my chats with Marj when I returned to Syracuse from my times in the field, and it was always a pleasure to approach data analysis through the prism of Marj's keen ethnographic eye. Elizabeth Clifford gave me insightful feedback and, through the years, has invited me to workshop the data from this project with the brilliant student participants in her immigration seminar at Towson University.

I am grateful for the institutional support and resources I received from the Connecticut State University–American Association of University Professors Research grants that allowed for data collection and transcription support beyond the dissertation. I gratefully acknowledge a publication subvention from the University of Connecticut Humanities Institute Book Support Award. A Carnegie African Diaspora Fellowship allowed me to engage in intellectual conversations with colleagues in Ghana, and I benefitted from insightful feedback from a public lecture I gave based on the book project. I had the opportunity to participate in several other workshops and conferences where I received feedback that helped advance the project. Some of these workshops and conversations include the biennial conferences organized by the Carework Network; a Gender and Migration workshop at University of California Irvine (UCI) organized by Katharine Donato, Cheryl Llewelyn, and Laura Enriquez; and a Care and Gender Migration conference at Humboldt University in Berlin, Germany. At Humboldt, I had the honor of meeting migration scholar extraordinaire Rhacel Parrenãs. She gave me a set of comments in Berlin and followed through with mentorship that helped sharpen my thinking around class, social mobility, and gender among migrant care workers. Thanks to Rhacel for showing me that the distant intellectual giants who shape our thinking and trajectories in graduate school can be even more generous and kind mentors in real life.

Some of the quoted material and argument in chapter 2 is reprinted with the permission of Cambridge Scholars Publishing. Additionally, some of the material in chapter 4 appeared in print in the article "Learning to Care: Work Experiences and Identity Formation among African Immigrant Care Workers," *International Journal of Care and Caring* 2, no. 1: 7–25 and is reproduced with the permission of Bristol University Press through PLSclear.

I owe a debt of gratitude to Rutgers University Press for bringing this book to completion. I want to thank Mignon Duffy, Kim Price-Glynn, and Amy Armenia for their support. I am deeply indebted to Mignon for introducing me to care work scholarship and for her support of my work and early development as a scholar. I thank Mignon, Kim, and Amy for their enthusiastic support for this book, their insightful feedback on drafts of the manuscript, and for developing the series in which it has found its home. I also want to thank Mary Johnson Osirim, who also read drafts of the book. Their close readings and focused attention helped me sharpen my arguments and highlight the book's contributions. I thank Peter Mickulas, my editor at Rutgers, for his enthusiastic support of the book. His gentle kindness assured me that my voice and, more importantly, the voice of my research subjects was valued.

This book bears the intellectual mark of many of my colleagues. At Central Connecticut State University, John O'Connor, Fiona Pearson, Heather Rodriguez, Christina Barmon, Beth Merenstein, and Bruce Day gave me useful feedback on early articles that inform this book. I am thankful for the support of my colleagues at the University of Connecticut (UConn). In particular, Andrew Deener kindly read the book proposal and gave me insightful comments on sample chapters. Bandana Purkayastha and Manisha Desai continue to provide models for integrity in leadership and excellence in scholarship and have been excellent mentors. Both constantly checked on the progress of my writing and gave me much-needed advice, encouragement, and support. Melina Pappademos and my colleagues in Africana Studies have provided a stimulating and nourishing intellectual home.

At Syracuse University, I found comrades who would become great friends as well as fellow travelers in my academic journey. They have each believed in me, inspired me by their brilliance and accomplishments, and provided companionship and friendship when I needed them most. Many of them are still key interlocuters with whom I continue to share the joys and travails of academia. I am grateful for the friendship and colleagueship of Mellony Manning Banyikwa, Ynesse Abdul-Malak, Tre Wentling, Natalee Simpson, Andrew Banyikwa, Ian Brown, and Kimberly Williams Brown. Kim offered me the use of her parent's beautiful home in Mandeville, Jamaica, in the summer of 2021. As a result, I had the luxury of spending six glorious weeks in splendid (semi) isolation, where I worked on bringing this book into the world. For the writing retreat and respite when I needed it, and for giving me the push that brought this book to its conclusion, I will forever be grateful to Kim and her family. I also am grateful to Kim for our many phone conversations in which we have exchanged stimulating ideas.

Chidi Blyden Rowe provided me with housing in Washington, DC, at various points as I conducted the research. She was a fun housemate and has maintained a friendship and interest in the project and in my career. Other friends I met while on the tenure track inspired me with their own books and offered me advice and support. They include Daisy Reyes, Ivan Small, Marguerite Nguyen, and Dann Broyld. Ilara Mahdi, Juanita Ceesay, and Sophronia Lewis have been lifelong friends and have provided me laughter and levity when I needed it most. Our memories of our childhoods in Sierra Leone provide a much-needed bridge between my past and my present. I also am grateful to Kasandre and Adly Nestor, friends I made in Connecticut who supported me in those first lonely years in a new place and graciously included me as the infamous "third wheel" on many of their dates and activities.

I am extremely fortunate to be part of a large West African family, and to have married into an equally large Nigerian and African American family. These bonds of blood and love span continents (Africa, Europe, United States). The list would be too long were I to mention everyone by name, but needless to say, I often have felt supported and grounded by the love of my clan. I am fortunate to count among my family members the erudite historian of the African Diaspora and U.S. immigration Violet Showers Johnson. I thank Auntie Iyabo, as she is fondly known in our family, for paving the way for my journey to the United States and for making it possible for me to attend Agnes Scott College, where she started her career. I am grateful to her, her husband, Percy Johnson, and their son, Percy Johnson Jr. (PJ), who welcomed me into their home for my first four years in the United States. I thank Auntie Iyabo also for her continued support and mentorship. Her scholarship, astute observations, and insights helped shape the book for the better. I thank all my aunts and uncles, as well as cousins who have nurtured and supported me from my childhood to this day. Una all tenki, tenki.

My deep gratitude goes to my parents, Moses and Adeliza Showers, who have taught me that a sound intellectual mind must also be a kind and compassionate one. They have modeled through their achievements, sacrifices, humility, grace, and service to others the kind of life I will be most fortunate to achieve. Their bottomless and unconditional faith in me has helped me surmount many a challenge. Their love, support, and sacrifice helped me cross the finish line in graduate school and provided some of the material and emotional sustenance that allowed me to undertake the research for this book. I also thank my brothers Dandeson and Adewale and my sister-in-law Martha for their love and support, and my nephew and niece, Micah and Malaika, for always reminding me that thinking, learning, and creating new things can be full of joy.

I am thankful to my husband, Ilesanmi Adeboye, whom I had the life-changing good fortune to meet just after completing the final round of fieldwork for this book. Ilesanmi has been my most ardent supporter and a source of deep personal happiness. From helping to refine the book's central arguments to brainstorming titles to reading elements of the book, his love, patience, kindness, and intellect have sustained me and, in the process, transformed him into the best mathematician-sociologist partner and friend. He injected optimism and positivity in the low points, and his patience never wavered. For providing me with a safe, loving, supportive, and intellectually stimulating home and family life, I thank Ilesanmi. I also thank my parents-in-law, Adeniran and Barbara Adeboye, for showing a keen interest in the arguments of the book and the process of writing it. Their commitment to, and soul-enriching conversations around, the global Black world continue to provide inspiration. Lastly, I am grateful to the entire Adeboye/Neverdon family for their love and support.

NOTES

INTRODUCTION

1. See appendix B for description of nursing jobs.

2. The Washington, DC, Office of Disability Services uses the term "direct support professional" to describe a segment of the health care labor force that provides hands-on care, such as feeding, bathing, and help with mobility for adults with physical and intellectual disabilities.

3. According to the Washington, DC, Office of Disability Services, QIDPs are "responsible for integrating, coordinating and monitoring each client's active treatment. They are staff: (a) who possess at least one year of experience working directly with persons with intellectual disabilities or other developmental disabilities; (b) who are either a physician and surgeon, or a[n] osteopathy physician and surgeon, a registered nurse, or a human services professional possessing at least a bachelor's degree in a human services field, including but not limited to sociology, special education, rehabilitation counseling or psychology."

4. Racialization is the way people and groups are absorbed into hierarchical racial systems by racial assignment and categorization.

5. I use the term "direct care work" as the umbrella term to refer to the paraprofessional occupational categories that involve care for the elderly, sick, and disabled in institutional and home settings. It includes the hands-on care work performed by HHAs, CNAs, and DSPs. I use the term "health care work" to broadly refer to the work of direct care workers as well as other health care professionals such as LPNs, RNs, NPs, and managers/administrators with supervisory roles.

6. According to Jeanne Batalova of the Migration Policy Institute, "Health-care support occupations were expected to grow the fastest among the 22 broad workforce-wide occupational groups analyzed by the U.S. Bureau of Labor Statistics (BLS), with home health care and home care as well as institutional care projected to increase by 18 percent, followed by health-care practitioners and technical occupations (12 percent). These projections were before the shifts in the labor market starting in 2020, because of the COVID-19 disruptions to daily life."

7. Health care occupations employed approximately 14.7 million native-born and immigrant workers in 2018, up from 12 million in 2010. Pre-COVID-19 health care occupations were projected to account for 1.9 million of the 8.4 million jobs expected to be newly created in the United States between 2018 and 2028 (Batalova 2020).

8. The term "foreign born" refers to people residing in the United States at the time of the Census survey who were not U.S. citizens at birth. The foreign-born population includes naturalized citizens, lawful permanent residents (LPRs), refugees and asylees, legal nonimmigrants (including those on student, work, or certain other temporary visas), and persons residing in the country without authorization. This book uses the terms "immigrant" and "foreign born" interchangeably. The terms "U.S. born" and "native born" are used interchangeably and refer to persons with U.S. citizenship at birth, including persons born in Puerto Rico or abroad born to a U.S.-citizen parent.

9. Among the 14.7 million workers employed in health care occupations in 2018, 2.6 million (18 percent) were foreign born. Relative to their share of the total workforce, immigrants make up disproportionate shares among both high-end professional- and lower-tiered paraprofessional health care workers. For example, immigrants accounted for 28 percent of the

958,000 physicians and surgeons practicing in the United States, and 38 percent of the 492,000 home health aides. (Batalova 2020).

10. I selected Nigeria, Ghana, Sierra Leone, and Liberia—four of the top sending countries from West Africa in the Washington, DC, metro area that are also English speaking (Lorenzi and Batalova 2022). I included English-speaking Cameroonians (a country located in West Central Africa with English- and French-speaking populations) because of snowball sampling. Participants introduced me to a few co-workers who were Cameroonian. While selecting distinct national groups, I do not intend to construct a typology of migration patterns that are distinct to the national groups or to make specific claims about distinctive patterns among these groups. Instead, this book sheds light on recurring characteristics common among the population of West Africans in this area.

CHAPTER 1   MOVING TO AMERICA

1. For example, the Washington, DC, department of health requires that each new applicant for licensure, registration, or certification obtain a criminal background check. The policy states: "A criminal background check shall be conducted in accordance with States' and Metropolitan Police Department's (MPD) and the Federal Bureau of Investigation's (FBI) policies and procedures and in an FBI-approved environment, by means of fingerprinting and National Criminal Information Center checks and procedures. The FBI criminal background check shall disclose any criminal history of the prospective applicant over a seven (7) year period, in all jurisdictions within which the prospective applicant has worked or resided. The MPD shall conduct a similar criminal background check for offenses within the district," https://dchealth.dc.gov/service/criminal-background-check.

2. Deferred Action for Childhood Arrivals, DACA, is a policy enacted by President Obama through an executive branch memorandum. This policy allows for some undocumented immigrants brought to the United States as children to apply for and receive a renewable two-year period of reprieve from deportation and to become eligible for a work permit. To qualify, recipients have to meet minimum educational requirements and cannot have felonies or serious misdemeanors on their records. See Roberto Gonzales (2016) *Lives in Limbo: Undocumented and Coming of Age in America,* for an in-depth look into the lives and experiences of undocumented youth.

3. On January 4, 1979, there was a coup d'état led by the late Flight Lieutenant Jerry J. Rawlings, who later became the president of Ghana.

4. The 1980 Refugee Act aligned U.S. immigration law with the international standards set in the 1951 Geneva Convention, which defines refugees as people outside their country of residence and unable to return due to a well-founded fear of persecution due to race, religion, nationality, membership in a particular social group, or political opinion (UNHCR 2010).

5. Liberia has had political instability since 1980 (Arthur 2009), when Sergeant Samuel K. Doe overthrew the government of President William Tolbert, ending the more than one-hundred-year rule of the True Whig Party. Doe subsequently presided over a period of turmoil in Liberia marked by ethnic divisions, allegations of corruption, and brutality. Charles Taylor overthrew Doe in 1990 after a rebel insurgency that lasted about seven years. Hundreds of thousands of people in Liberia were killed, injured, or displaced from their homes. The conflict left the country in economic shambles. Liberian insurgents then formed the United Liberation Movement of Liberia Democracy (ULIMO). Based in Sierra Leone, ULIMO waged a war of opposition against Taylor's National Patriotic Front of Liberia that lasted several years. Many Liberian refugees fled during this period. In the meantime, constant skirmishes and uprisings and a stagnant economy created desperation. Taylor also interfered in

the affairs of the other countries in the region. He armed and supported the Revolutionary United Front (RUF), a group that also waged a long uprising and rebellion in Sierra Leone that culminated when the RUF joined forces with the Armed Forces Revolutionary Council (ARFC), a group made of up members of the army. Together, the AFRC and RUF overthrew the democratically elected government in Sierra Leone in May 1997. This action, as well as the long-standing rebellion that had been ongoing in parts of the country, also cost the lives of hundreds of thousands; many Sierra Leoneans lost their homes and belongings; families were separated; and thousands more sought refuge in other countries (Arthur, 2000, 2009). Charles Taylor, the former Head of State of Liberia, was convicted in April 2012 by the International Criminal Court in The Hague of aiding and abetting war crimes through his support for armed militias and rebels in Sierra Leone. Today, both Liberia and Sierra Leone have instituted democratically elected governments and have reported relative calm and stability. Both countries have seen economic growth in recent years and have made tremendous strides in recovering from the ravages of war. However, poverty and unemployment remain dire challenges for the resilient populace of this country. Both countries, together with Guinea, were ravaged by an outbreak of the Ebola Virus disease that killed over 11,000 people between 2014 and 2016.

6. Liberians were granted TPS from 1991 to 2017. Likewise, Sierra Leoneans were eligible for TPS at different periods from 1999 to 2017. A country's nationals are granted TPS due to conditions in the country that temporarily prevent them from returning safely or in certain circumstances where the country is unable to handle the return of its nationals adequately, usually because of armed conflict or environmental disaster. The designation comes from the Department of Homeland Security, and grantees are allowed temporary work permits, which they can hold for as long as the designation remains.

7. The most popular form of this visa is the H1B visa, which is a category for specialty occupations. Specialty occupations usually require at least a bachelor's degree. The employer must prove that the foreign worker has a particular specialized skill that makes their employment necessary and that there was no U.S. worker at the same skill level and expertise who could perform those functions. These employment provisions in immigration law also are gendered and result in systematic disadvantage of women since women are less likely than men to qualify based on skills valued in the labor market (see, for example, Banerjee 2022, 2018).

8. I did not find striking differences between the men and women in this study in terms of mode of entry into the United States. Men and women entered the United States via similar pathways: on student or tourist visas, as family-sponsored migrants, diversity visa lottery winners, or refugees. While some women, such as Henricia discussed in this chapter, entered the United States as "dependents" of their husbands who had entered the United States on student visas, there were some women, such as Yenoh, who came as independent migrants on student or other visas, as did some men. While men were more likely to be primary migrants, there were women, such as Harriet, who were primary migrants who left their husbands behind, with those husbands joining them later. Other women and men migrated as single people, with some meeting and marrying their spouses in the United States. See Banerjee, *The Opportunity Trap: High-Skilled Workers, Indian Families, and the Failures of the Dependent Visa Program* for a fuller analysis of the gendered consequences of ostensibly gender-neutral immigration policies. Banerjee focused on two groups of labor migrants: female nurses who migrated as primary migrants and their husbands, who migrated as dependents of their visas; and male IT workers and their "dependent" wives. This study design of focusing on two groups of workers in gender-segmented labor markets allowed for a comparative analysis of gendered differences within divergent spheres. See, also, Gowayed, *Refuge: How the State Shapes Human Potential* for a more detailed discussion of how gender shapes the incorporation of refugees in

the United States and the divergent labor market experiences of men and women. Unlike my participants, who had equal labor force participation rates prior to migration, in Gowayed's study, many women had not worked outside the home. Thus, for these women, migration opened some opportunities for work in the public sphere that they lacked back home. Like other classical studies of gender and migration have shown (see, for example, Sylvia Pedraza, 1991, *Women and Migration: The Social Consequences of Gender*), migration can open new opportunities for work outside the home, access to wages, etc., which can prove emancipatory for some women. For my female participants who had not only been active in the labor market but were in professional or high-status occupations prior to migration, migration to the United States was not "freeing." Men and women, therefore, in this book had largely similar experiences of downward mobility and labor market displacement upon migration.

CHAPTER 2   PATHWAYS AND ENTRYWAYS INTO CARE

1. Immigrant pioneers are the first individuals or groups to settle in a particular area in a host land. Often, they pave the way for the migration of others and their entry into specific labor niches through the activation of social networks that connect their homeland and host lands. See Bashi (2007), Dhingra (2012), and Poros (2011) for a description of the role of these immigrant pioneers. I build on these understandings of immigrant pioneers in my conceptualization of "care pioneers." Care pioneers are immigrant care workers who first made inroads into care occupations. They then encouraged members of their immigrant kin and other social networks to become care workers, either by directly asking them to enter the field or by modeling an image of success that then compels others to join the workforce. They also informally brokered jobs in the "gray market" for care or more formally through their health care recruitment and provision businesses.

2. See Miraftab, *Global Heartland: Displaced Labor, Transnational Lives and Local Placemaking* for a contrasting case study of French-speaking West Africans with legalized immigration statuses and similar premigration high human capital who worked in meat-packing plants because those jobs did not require English language skills. Miraftab's respondents had large extended families and familial obligations and debts, sometimes incurred to facilitate their travel to the United States, which forced them to stay in "dirty jobs" in the meat-packing industry. Though they remitted significant amounts to family members back home, my respondents did not articulate having any such debts that would tie them to low status, low prestige occupations. See, also, Stoller (2001), *Money has no Smell: The Africanization of New York City* for an ethnography on French-speaking West Africans who worked as informal street vendors in New York City.

CHAPTER 3   THE BUSINESS OF CARE

1. This pseudonym (with title) captures how this participant was referenced by her employers and her children. Addressing her as Mrs. Johnson throughout this chapter is also in keeping with cultural norms of respect for community elders as well as to reflect the regard in which she was held by the Sierra Leonean immigrant community in that area.

2. This is a pseudonym. I have used pseudonyms for two of the businesses named in this chapter.

3. At the time of my research, the age range of their care recipients was from twenty-one years old to ninety-four years old.

4. According to Washington, DC, DDS, "Day habilitation services are aimed at developing activities and skills acquisition to support or further integrate community opportunities outside of a person's home and assist the person in developing a full life within the community. Day habilitation services are aimed at developing meaningful adult activities and skills acquisition to: support or further community integration, inclusion, and exploration, improve communication skills; improve or maintain physical, occupational and/or speech and language functional skills; foster independence, self-determination and self-advocacy and autonomy; support people to build and maintain relationships; facilitate the exploration of employment and/or integrated retirement opportunities; help a person achieve valued social roles; and to foster and encourage people on their pathway to community integration, employment and the development of a full life in the person's community." Also, "Residential Habilitation Service is provided by an agency in a licensed home serving four to six persons that is owned or leased and operated by the agency. Residential Habilitation is a blended service that provides habilitation, personal care, nursing, other residential supports, and transportation to the persons living in the home."

5. Asset limits are $2,000 for an individual and $3,000 for a couple (Osterman 2017). An administrator at Worldwide confirmed these amounts for their population of care recipients.

6. Since this research was conducted over the summer months spread over a few years, I found that a couple of the businesses with whom I had made initial contact were defunct when I returned to the field in subsequent visits. The office spaces were occupied by non-healthcare businesses on those return visits. In general, my observations about a small minority of the agencies were that they were run by unscrupulous characters with dubious employment practices. One scene I witnessed occurred in the summer of 2012. I paid a visit to the office of an agency whose owner I had met previously. On this visit, I noticed a group of home care workers gathered in the hallways, while the main door to the office was shut with no sign of activity going on. The workers, all Black women in scrubs, their distress obvious, stated loudly and aggressively that they had come to receive paychecks for the prior week's work. The managers and administrators were nowhere to be found. The scene was very chaotic, and amid the shouts and commotion, I could decipher that it was not unusual. Fly-by-night operations and wage theft seemed to be part of the story of a few of these businesses. Since my focus was on the establishment of health care businesses and the experience of care workers and not necessarily on the labor practices or labor relations of these companies, I did not delve further into these matters. But as exemplified by Worldwide and the other businesses featured in this chapter, most African-owned businesses I encountered were legitimate, ethical, and run by people for whom I came to develop a lot of respect and admiration.

7. According to the Washington, DC, DOH, "A Home care agency means an agency, organization or distinct part thereof, other than a hospice, that provides either directly or through a contractual agreement, a program of health care, habilitative or rehabilitative therapy, personal care services, homemaker services, chore services or other supportive services to sick individuals or individuals with disabilities living at home or in a community residence facility."

8. Assisted living facilities are designed to grant their residents independent living conditions as a contrasting living experience to nursing homes. Assisted living facilities provide residents assistance with ADLS but, unlike nursing homes, do not provide complex medical services. There are also no health-specific entrance requirements. People in assisted living are generally less sick and require less help with ADLs than people in nursing homes but are generally in worse health than the rest of the population (Osterman 2017).

9. A certificate of need demonstrates a public need for the new facility or entity. To obtain this certificate, the applicant first submits a letter of intent to the state (or District) DOH,

which provides information on the location of the proposed facility and a description of the facility type. Then the applicant issues a public notice (advertisement) in a paper with a local circulation and attends a pre-application conference with relevant staff. In DC, applicants pay $5,000 or 3 percent of the proposed capital expenditure, whichever is greater, up to $300,000. https://dchealth.dc.gov/node/160472.

10. I have used pseudonyms to characterize interactions where the full names of clients were used.

11. Service coordinators acted as a liaison between DDS and other members of the care recipient's service team. They made sure individuals were eligible for services through DDS. Working within a person-centered framework, they discussed the individuals' needs and goals (e.g., day program attendance, employment preferences) and connected them to the appropriate service providers.

CHAPTER 4   DISABILITY SUPPORT

1. While this was my observation of the training of disability support professionals at Worldwide, other accounts of HHA or CNA training differ considerably. These reports show instruction in the practical and physical aspects of care. For instance, Richard Schweid (2021) reports lessons in bathing clients; safety, and infection control; observing, recording, and reporting changes in clients' condition; and strategies for effectively caring for patients with Alzheimer's disease.

2. Employees at Worldwide referred to the older nurses with the title "nurse" followed by last name or first name. Younger nurses in their thirties and forties were simply referenced by their first names, as were the VP of the company, the DON, and the lead staff trainer and recruitment coordinator (the middle-aged children of the company owners). Since there were relatively few nurses on staff compared to DSPs, and even fewer nurses addressed by the title "nurse," to maintain confidentiality, I have not assigned a specific pseudonym to this particular nurse.

3. BLS data by occupation is derived from the National Compensation Survey, Occupational Employment Survey, or the Current Population Survey which provide updated data in intercensus years. The most updated data available at the time of this book's writing was for 2018.

CHAPTER 5   PATIENT-PROVIDER INTERACTIONS AND PROFESSIONAL IDENTITIES IN NURSING

1. Much of the coverage in the Western media sensationalized the epidemic. Television and print media reports and images graphically portrayed Black African deaths and suffering and utilized racist tropes to discuss backward "cultural practices," such as consuming "bush meat," and the population's ignorance and distrust of biomedicine and health institutions that supposedly perpetuated the crisis. Articles with sensationalist headlines appeared in major global media outlets such as CNN, the *Washington Post*, and the Associated Press as well as more local publications. Examples of such headlines include: "Ebola Outbreak in West Africa Now the Worst in History," https://mashable.com/2014/06/17/ebola-outbreak-interactive-data -visualization/; "This is the Worst Ebola Outbreak in History: Here's Why You Should be Worried," https://www.washingtonpost.com/news/worldviews/wp/2014/07/28/this-is-the -worst-ebola-outbreak-in-history-heres-why-you-should-be-worried/; "Why an Ebola Epidemic is Spinning Out of Control," https://www.cnn.com/2014/07/24/opinion/garrett-ebola /index.html; "2 Americans Infected with Ebola in Liberia Coming to Atlanta Hospital,"

https://www.cnn.com/2014/08/01/health/ebola-outbreak/; "Ebola Outbreak in West Africa Aided by Ignorance and Distrust," https://guardianlv.com/2014/07/ebola-outbreak-in-west -africa-aided-by-ignorance-and-distrust-says-who/; and "Fear of Ebola Breeds a Terror of Doctors," https://www.nytimes.com/2014/07/28/world/africa/ebola-epidemic-west-africa -guinea.html. Other commentary, especially on social media platforms such as Twitter, was more critical and called out the explicit racism and bias in the mainstream media coverage. Counter headlines analyzed the situation from a point of view of wealth and income inequality between global north and global south; white privilege and the nexus with medial humani-tarianism; and the ongoing disregard for Black lives globally. An example of these head-lines is "Why Do Two White Americans get the Ebola Serum, while Hundreds of Africans Die?," https://www.washingtonpost.com/posteverything/wp/2014/08/06/why-do-two -white-americans-get-the-ebola-serum-while-hundreds-of-africans-die/. A tweet from twit-ter handle The Public Archive reads: "Ebola Serum Given to White Christian Aid Workers, while Black African Heathen Die," with an accompanying link to this *LA Times* article: https://www.latimes.com/science/sciencenow/la-sci-sn-ebola-serum-20140804-story.html. Another tweet from a since-suspended twitter account read: "2 Whites Gets Ebola and are Put on 'Experimental' Drugs. Africans Die in Huge Numbers. Old story. Blacks Lives Don't Matter."

2. Other studies situated in the United States, Canada, and Europe also have found that, in addition to racial discrimination, Black African immigrants are subject to a specific form of discrimination tied to their ethnic identities as people with recent migration histories from Africa (Creese 2011, 2019; Showers 2015a, 2015b; Tesfai 2021, 2020; Thomas 2014). This specific form of discrimination tied to African origin takes place in various contexts and settings, for example, work and the labor market (Tesfai 2021, 2020; Tesfai and Thomas 2020; Veit and Thijsen 2021) and schools and other educational institutions (Beoku-Betts 2004; Beoku-Betts and Njambi 2005). Among these, qualitative studies have revealed that Black African immi-grants perceive discrimination due to their ethnic origins in addition to their racial identities and status as immigrants. Quantitative studies have revealed disadvantages that accrue to African immigrants based on their race and ethnicity, with discrimination as one possible explanation for these inequalities.

3. This is a pseudonym. In keeping with the general trend of using pseudonyms in this book, I chose a traditional Nigerian/Yoruba last name to reflect the nationality and ethnicity of this nurse participant.

4. For instance, high-pressure, skilled areas such as the intensive care unit were described as attracting mostly white nurses, and Africans were thought to be concentrated in nursing homes that required attending to less pleasant personal care and other mundane duties.

5. Most of the foundational studies on this issue were qualitative in nature and drew from the experiences of mostly English-speaking Caribbean immigrants residing in New York City and extrapolated from these findings to make universal claims about Black immigrant groups.

6. See Tod Hamilton (2019) *Immigration and the Remaking of Black America* for a full discus-sion of these debates around whether culture, immigrant selectivity, or favorable contexts of reception versus racism are factors that explain better outcomes for immigrant Blacks in com-parison to African Americans. See Hamilton, also, for a discussion of disparities in earnings, home ownership, and other measures among immigrant Blacks and African Americans.

7. The theories of sociologist Eduardo Bonilla-Silva (2004) provide a more nuanced under-standing of why these strategies fail. Bonilla-Silva theorizes a tripartite racial categorization system in the United States, comprising whites and a collective black category alongside an intermediate category he calls "honorary whites." The honorary white category comprises "well-off Mexicans and Hispanics, certain Asian groups such as Koreans and the Chinese, and

American Indians who do not live on reservations." Upwardly mobile members of these groups can become "whitened" or at least approximate the benefits of whiteness. However, many Black groups, because of their skin color and pervasive anti-Blackness in the United States, cannot become "honorary whites," even as they become upwardly mobile. Attempts to assimilate through strategies such as professional distancing prove shortsighted and do little to dismantle racial occupational barriers and structures and may, in fact, perpetuate them.

CHAPTER 6   NURSING A PATHWAY TO THE AMERICAN DREAM

1. See Pawan Dhingra, *Life Behind the Lobby: Indian American Motel Owners and the American Dream*, for an example that critically engages the success of an immigrant group within this framework of the American dream. See Zulema Valdez, *The New Entrepreneurs: How Race, Class and Gender Shape American Enterprise* and *Entrepreneurs and The Search for the American Dream*, for an analysis that shatters the "myth" of the American dream, focusing on inequalities and constraints faced by immigrant minority entrepreneurs.

2. According to the BLS, the average yearly wage for a registered nurse in 2020 was $71,870 in Virginia, $77,910 in Maryland, and $94,9820 for the District of Columbia.

3. Cati Coe (2019) documented the changes to the Fair Labor Standards Act, FLSA, that mandated overtime wages for home care workers who had previously been excluded from FLSA provisions. These changes meant that, starting in 2016, home care workers in Washington, DC, were eligible for overtime compensation for work exceeding forty hours a week. Data for this study was collected prior to these changes, so study participants who had worked as home care workers were not eligible for overtime pay. However, most of the direct care workers in this study routinely worked sixty to eighty hours a week, and did so by combining employers, not necessarily through accruing overtime compensation with one employer.

4. Employees at Worldwide referred to the older nurses with the title "nurse" followed by last name or first name. Younger nurses in their thirties and forties were simply referenced by their first names, as were the VP of the company, the DON, and the lead staff trainer and recruitment coordinator (the middle-aged children of the company owners). Since there were relatively few nurses on staff compared to DSPs, and even fewer nurses addressed by the title "nurse," to maintain confidentiality, I have not assigned a specific pseudonym to this nurse.

5. To objectively assess the value and worth of homes I visited, I reviewed some housing records publicly available at www.realtor.com, a home value resource. Realtor.com does not provide the name or any identifying information about the current or previous owner of properties. The website lists the current value of the home (at the time of the book's writing), the year the home was last recorded as sold, and the appreciation or depreciation value. Information about the last purchase year allowed me to estimate the worth of the home at the time I conducted interviews and confirmed whether the home was under the same ownership as when I conducted the research. In all but one case, the records showed that the home was owned by the same person(s) as at the time of my research. In all cases, the homes had appreciated in value over the years from purchase to current year, with the appreciation values ranging from a low of $34,830 for a house last sold in 2005 to a staggering high of $338,301 for a home last sold in 1986. Adjusted home values for select single-family homes owned by African nurses at time of purchase are as follows: $601,400; $575,000; $537,7000; and $131,000 (this last was purchased in 1986 and had appreciated by $338,301). Home sizes were, on average, between 3,500 and 4,000 square feet. All these homes were in Montgomery and Prince George's counties in Maryland, except for one that was in Virginia.

6. Records show that one of these houses was purchased in 1986.

7. Townhomes were worth less than the single-family homes; two I looked up had sold for $204,680 and $350,000, respectively.

8. This was an exceptional year in which she had worked many overtime hours. Kate estimated her average yearly salary at $120,000, still far above the average salary for RNs in that region and nationally.

9. In a follow-up interview conducted in 2021, an administrator at Worldwide reported the following wages for their staff: QIDPs, $60,000 per annum; house managers, $47,000 per annum; DSPs $15.40 per hour. In addition, she stated that they provided financial bonuses twice a year and a cost-of-living wage increase every year. They provided additional benefits, health insurance (mandated by the Affordable Care Act, ACA since 2015), and a life insurance benefit policy valued at $50,000.

10. The reality of working for coethnics in ethnic enterprises has been debated in immigration scholarship. Some scholars view ethnic enterprises as providing a path of upward mobility outside of the primary labor market, whereas others have called attention to exploitation that can occur in these settings (Portes and Bach 1985; Sanders and Nee 1996). While some West African administrators of health care businesses registered some discontent with coethnics (for example, they complained about the lack of perceived professionalism of their staff who took advantage of their ethnic and familial ties and connections), the workers did not discuss any dissatisfaction with wages or the terms and conditions of their employment. It is possible that these workers may have not felt comfortable disclosing those kinds of grievances with me. In my interactions at Worldwide, however, I noticed a spirit of ethnic camaraderie as well as professionalism. Workers generally spoke to each other in Krio, the Sierra Leonean lingua franca, in informal interactions; they joked around with each other during breaks and brought in local dishes for lunch. But in conducting business, English was generally spoken, and employees conducted themselves as one would expect in any business.

11. https://awcaa.org.

12. See, for example, Vivian Louie, *Keeping the Immigrant Bargain: The Costs and Rewards of Success in America.*

13. Hyper-selection "refers to a dual positive selectivity where the immigrant group, on average, is more educated than the national average in their country of destination and more educated than the national average in their country of origin" (Lee and Zhou 2015, 6).

CONCLUSION

1. In July 2021, a criminal complaint filed in Baltimore, Maryland, charged two African immigrants for conspiring with a third person to "commit health care fraud, conspiracy to commit false statements relating to health care matters, and false statements to health care matters, in connection with a scheme to produce and sell fraudulent nursing transcripts and diplomas." See https://www.justice.gov/usao-md/pr/three-individuals-facing-federal-charges-participating -healthcare-fraud-scheme-sell.

AFTERWORD

1. In May 2020, a piece on African immigrant care workers in Minnesota was published in an independent digital newspaper dedicated to news about immigrants and communities of color in that state. See https://sahanjournal.com/immigration/in-healthcare-work-african-immigrants -feel-brunt-of-covid-19/. This publication in a niche journal focusing on one geography was, to

the best of my knowledge, the only news media article dedicated to African immigrant care workers in the first wave of the coronavirus.

2. https://www.sba.gov/funding-programs/loans/covid-19-relief-options/paycheck-protection-program.

3. https://awcaa.org/our-team/aisha-deen/.

APPENDIX A

1. I recruited all participants in this study in person. Other recruitment strategies approved by my university's Institutional Review Board, such as posting flyers soliciting participants in West African-owned businesses such as grocery stores or emailing recruitment letters to agency administrators did not yield any results.

2. These lists were public records obtainable from the Washington, DC, Department of Health website. They contained the names of agencies that were contracted as official providers for the DC DOH. Each agency listed a contact person. To determine African-owned/managed agencies, I picked names that were recognizable to me as African in origin. I expanded my access through snowball sampling methods as my initial contacts referred me to other African-owned agencies in their networks. There were some limitations with this method. By drawing from a DOH resource, I also was limited to agencies that provided home care as opposed to other types of support, and that catered to Medicaid recipients. By relying solely on my judgment as to the ethnicity of contact persons, there was the possibility of misrecognition. It also was possible that the contact persons were paid employees, not owners of businesses. However, since no established databases identify the racial or ethnic makeup of long-term care and other health business owners, this was the most appropriate technique to come close to a systematic sample of African-owned or administered businesses. While not foolproof, this method was effective, as all the agencies I approached were, indeed, African-owned. I gained access to the disability support agencies through snowball sampling as care workers told me about agencies to which they were connected.

3. A Hoyer lift is a mobility tool used to help individuals with mobility challenges. Named for its inventor, the Hoyer lift is a portable total body lift, a patient lift used to help the individual get out of bed or bath, for instance. These devices can be freestanding, on wheels, or secured to a wall or ceiling, depending on the user's needs and room set-up.

REFERENCES

Adepoju, Aderanti. 2000. "Trends in International Migration from Africa." In *International Migration: Prospects and Policies in a Global Market*, edited by D. S. Massey and J. E. Taylor, 15–34. New York: Oxford University Press.

———. 2001. "Regional Organizations and Intra-Regional Migration in Sub-Saharan Africa: Challenges and Prospects." *International Migration* 39 (6): 43–60.

———. 2002. "Fostering Free Movement of Persons in West Africa: Achievements, Constraints and Prospects for Intraregional Migration." *International Migration* 40 (2).

Aiken, Linda, and James Buchan. 2004. "Trends in International Nurse Migration." *Health Affairs* 23 (3): 69–77.

Alba, Richard, and Victor Nee. 2003. *Remaking the American Mainstream: Assimilation and Contemporary Immigration*. Cambridge, MA: Harvard University Press.

Altorjai, Szilvia, and Jeanne Batalova. 2017. "Immigrant Health Care Workers in the United States." Migration Information Source, Migration Policy Institute (June 28, 2017). http://www.migrationpolicy.org/article/immigrant-health-care-workers-united-states.

American Association of Colleges of Nursing. 2019. "Fact Sheet: Enhancing Diversity in the Nursing Profession." https://www.aacnnursing.org/Portals/42/News/Factsheets/Enhancing-Diversity-Factsheet.pdf.

American Association of Colleges of Nursing. 2020. "Fact Sheet: Nursing Shortage." https://www.aacnnursing.org/Portals/42/News/Factsheets/Nursing-Shortage-Factsheet.pdf.

Anderson, Monica. 2015. *A Rising Share of the U.S. Black Population Is Foreign Born*. Washington, DC: Pew Research Center. https://www.pewresearch.org/social-trends/2015/04/09/a-rising-share-of-the-u-s-black-population-is-foreign-born/.

Armstrong, Pat, and Hugh Armstrong. 2019. *The Privatization of Care: The Case of Nursing Homes*. New York: Routledge.

Aronson, Joshua, Diana Burgess, Sean M. Phelan, and Lindsay Juarez. 2013. "Unhealthy Interactions: The Role of Stereotype Threat in Health Disparities." *American Journal of Public Health* 103 (1): 50–56.

Arthur, John A. 2000. *Invisible Sojourners: African Immigrant Diaspora in the United States*. Westport, CT: Praeger.

———. 2009. *African Immigrant Women in the United States: Crossing Transnational Borders*. New York: Palgrave Macmillan.

Ayisi, Florence, and Catalyn Brylla. 2013. "The Politics of Representation and Audience Reception: Alternative Visions of Africa." *Research in African Literatures* 44 (2): 125–141.

Bakan, Abigail, and Daiva Stasiulis. 1995. "Making the Match: Domestic Placement Agencies and the Racialization of Women's Work." *Signs: Journal of Women in Culture and Society* 20 (2): 303–335.

Ball, Rochelle. 2004. "Divergent Development, Racialised Rights: Globalized Labour Markets and the Trade of Nurses—The Case of the Philippines." *Women's Studies International Forum* 27 (2): 119–133.

Banerjee, Pallavi. 2018. "Subversive Self-Employment: Intersectionality and Self-Employment among Dependent Visa Holders in the United States." *American Behavioral Scientist* 63 (2): 186–207.

————. 2022. *The Opportunity Trap: High-Skilled Workers, Indian Families, and the Failures of the Dependent Visa Program*. New York: New York University Press.

Bashi, Vilna. 2007. *Survival of the Knitted: Immigrant Social Networks in a Stratified World*. Stanford: Stanford University Press.

Batalova, Jeanne. 2018. "Immigrant Health-Care Workers in the United States." Migration Information Source, Migration Policy Institute. Retrieved October 15, 2020. https://www.migrationpolicy.org/article/immigrant-health-care-workers-united-states-2018.

Bennett, Pamela, and Amy Lutz. 2009. "How African American Is the Net Black Advantage? Differences in College Attendance among Immigrant Blacks, Native Blacks, and Whites." *Sociology of Education* 82 (1): 70–99.

Beoku-Betts, Josephine. 1994. "When Black Is Not Enough: Doing Field Research among Gullah Women." *NWSA Journal* 6 (3): 413–433.

————. 2004. "African Women Pursuing Graduate Studies in the Sciences: Racism, Gender Bias, and Third World Marginality." *NWSA Journal* 16 (1): 116–135.

Beoku-Betts, Josephine, and Warimu Njambi. 2005. "African Feminist Scholars in Women's Studies: Negotiating the Spaces of Transformation and Dislocation in the Study of Women." *Meridiens: Feminism, Race, Transnationalism* 6 (1): 113–132.

Bonilla-Silva, Eduardo. 2004. "From Bi-racial to Tri-racial: Towards a New System of Racial Stratification in the USA." *Ethnic and Racial Studies* 27 (6): 931–950.

Boris, Eileen, and Jennifer Klein. 2012. *Caring for America: Home Health Workers in the Shadow of the Welfare State*. Oxford: Oxford University Press.

Boris, Eileen, and Rhacel Parreñas, eds. 2010. *Intimate Labors: Cultures, Technologies, and the Politics of Care*. Stanford: Stanford University Press.

Brennan, Denise. 2004. *What's Love Got to Do with It: Transnational Desires and Sex Tourism in the Dominican Republic*. Durham: Duke University Press.

Brush, Barbara L., and Julie Sochalski. 2007. "International Nurse Migration: Lessons from the Philippines." *Policy, Politics & Nursing Practice* 8:37–46.

Buch, Elana D. 2018. *Inequalities of Aging: Paradoxes of Independence in American Home Care*. New York: New York University Press.

Buerhaus, Peter I., Douglas O. Staiger, and David I. Auerbach. 2003. "Is the Current Shortage of Hospital Nurses Ending?" *Health Affairs* 22 (6): 191–198.

Carty, Linda. 2003. "'Not a Nanny.' A Gendered, Transnational Analysis of Caribbean Domestic Workers in New York City." In *Decolonizing the Academy: African Diaspora Studies*, edited by C. Boyce-Davies, M. Gadsby, C. F. Peterson, and H. Williams. Trenton, NJ: Africa World Press.

Chambliss, Daniel F. 1996. *Beyond Caring: Hospitals, Nurses, and the Social Organization of Ethics*. Chicago: University of Chicago Press.

Chang, Grace. 2000. *Immigrant Women Workers in the Global Economy*. Cambridge, MA: South End Press.

Chapman, Susan, and Charlene Harrington. 2020. "Policies Matter! Factors Contributing to Nursing Home Outbreaks during the COVID-19 Pandemic." *Policy, Politics, & Nursing Practice* 21 (4): 191–192.

Chidambaram, Priya, Rachel Garfield, and Tricia Newman. 2020. "COVID-19 has Claimed the Lives of 100,000 Long-Term Care Residents and Staff." Kaiser Family Foundation. https://www.kff.org/policy-watch/covid-19-has-claimed-the-lives-of-100000-long-term-care-residents-and-staff/.

Choy, Ceniza. 2003. *Empire of Care: Nursing and Migration in Filipino American History*. Durham, NC: Duke University Press.

Cigler, Beverly A. 2021. "Nursing Homes and COVID-19: One State's Experience." *International Journal of Public Administration* 44 (11–12): 963–973.

Coe, Cati. 2019. *The New American Servitude: Political Belonging among African Immigrant Home Care Workers.* New York: New York University Press.

———. 2021. "African Immigrant Care Workers & COVID in the US: Their Fears, Protections, and Recalibrations" (February 16). http://somatosphere.net/2021/african-immigrant-care-workers-and-covid.html/.

Colen, Shelee. 1989. "'Just a Little Respect': West Indian Domestic Workers in New York City." In *Muchachas No More: Household Workers in Latin America and the Caribbean*, edited by E. Chaney and M. Garcia Castro. Philadelphia: Temple University Press.

———. 1990. "'Housekeeping for the Green Card': West Indian Household Workers, The State and Stratified Reproduction in New York." In *At Work in Homes: Household Workers in World Perspective*, edited by R. Sanjek and S. Colen. Washington, DC: American Anthropological Association.

———. 1995. "Like a Mother to Them: Stratified Reproduction and West Indian Child Care Workers and Employers in New York." In *Conceiving the New World Order: The Global Politics of Reproduction*, edited by F. D. Ginsburg and R. Rapp, 78–102. Berkeley: University of California Press.

Collins, Patricia Hill. 1991. *Black Feminist Thought: Knowledge, Consciousness, and the Politics of Empowerment.* New York: Routledge.

Conteh-Morgan, Earl, and Mac Dixon-Fyle. 1999. *Sierra Leone at the End of the Twentieth Century: History, Politics, and Society.* New York: Peter Lang.

Cottingham, Marci D. 2013. "Recruiting Men, Constructing Manhood: How Health Organizations Mobilize Masculinities as Nursing Recruitment Strategy." *Gender and Society* 28 (1): 133–156.

Covington-Ward, Yolanda. 2017. "African Immigrants in Low-Wage Direct Health Care: Motivations, Job Satisfaction, and Occupational Mobility." *Journal of Immigrant and Minority Health* 19 (3): 709–715.

Cranford, Cynthia. 2020. *Home Care Fault lines: Understanding Tensions and Creating Alliances.* Ithaca, NY: Cornell University Press.

Crawley, Heaven, and Dimitri Skleparis. 2018. "Refugees, Migrants, Neither, Both: Categorical Fetishism and the Politics of Bounding in Europe's 'Migration Crisis.'" *Journal of Ethnic and Migration Studies* 44 (1): 48–64.

Creese, Gillian. 2011. *The New African Diaspora in Vancouver: Immigration, Exclusion and Belonging.* Toronto: University of Toronto Press.

———. 2019. "'Where Are You From?' Racialization, Belonging and Identity among Second Generation African-Canadians." *Ethnic and Racial Studies* 42 (9): 1476–1494.

Dapremont, Jill. 2013. "A Review of Minority Recruitment and Retention Models Implemented in Undergraduate Nursing Programs." *Journal of Nursing Education and Practice* 43 (2): 112–119.

Degiuli, Francesca. 2011. "Labouring Lives: The Making of Home Eldercare Assistants in Italy." *Modern Italy* 16 (3): 45–61.

———. 2016. *Caring for a Living: Migrant Women, Aging Citizens and Italian Families.* London and New York: Oxford University Press.

Devault, Marjorie. 1999. "Talking and Listening from Women's Standpoint." In *Liberating Method: Feminism and Social Research*, 59–83. Philadelphia: Temple University Press.

Dhingra, Pawan. 2012. *Life behind the Lobby: Indian American Motel Owners and the American Dream.* Stanford: Stanford University Press.

Diamond, Timothy. 1992. *Making Gray Gold: Narratives of Nursing Home Care.* Chicago: University of Chicago Press.

Dodson, Lisa, and Rebekah Zincavage. 2007. "'It's Like a Family': Caring Labor, Exploitation and Race in Nursing Homes." *Gender and Society* 21(6): 905–928.

———. 2015. "'It's Like a Family': Caring Labor, Exploitation and Race in Nursing Homes." In *Caring on the Clock: The Complexities and Contradictions of Paid Care Work,* edited by M. Duffy, A. Armenia, and C. Stacey, 189–200. New Brunswick, NJ: Rutgers University Press.

Donkor, Martha. 2017. *The Experiences of Ghanaian Live-in Caregivers in the United States.* Lanham, MD: Lexington Books.

Dovlo, Delano. 2006. "Ghanaian Health Workers on the Causes and Consequences of Migration." In *Globalizing Migration Regimes,* edited by K. Tamas and J. Palme, 118–130. Aldershot, Hampshire: Ashgate.

Duffy, Mignon. 2005. "Reproducing Labor Inequalities: Challenges for Feminists Conceptualizing Care at the Intersections of Gender, Race, and Class." *Gender & Society* 19 (1): 66–82.

———. 2007. "Doing the Dirty Work: Gender, Race, and the Reproductive Labor in Historical Perspective, *Gender & Society* 21 (3): 313–336.

Duffy, Mignon, Amy Armenia, and Clare Stacey. 2015. "On the Clock, Off the Radar: Paid Care Work in the United States." In *Caring on the Clock: The Complexities and Contradictions of Paid Care Work,* edited by M. Duffy, A. Armenia, and C. Stacey, 3–13. New Brunswick, NJ: Rutgers University Press.

Durr, Marlene, and Adia Harvey Wingfield. 2011. "'Keep Your 'N' in Check!' African American Women and the Interactive Effects of Etiquette and Emotional Labor." *Critical Sociology* 37 (5): 557–571.

Dwyer, Rachel. E. 2013. "The Care Economy? Gender, Economic Restructuring, and Job Polarization in the U.S. Labor Market." *American Sociological Review* 78 (3): 390–416.

Eaton-Robb, Pat. 2021. "Nursing Schools See Applications Rise, Despite COVID Burnout." https://www.wcvb.com/article/nursing-schools-see-applications-rise-despite-covid -burnout/37961976#.

Echevarria-Estrada, Carlos, and Jeanne Batalova. 2019. "Sub-Saharan Africans in the United States." Migration Information Source, Migration Policy Institute. Retrieved October 10, 2020. https://www.migrationpolicy.org/article/sub-saharan-african-immigrants-united -states-2018.

Eckstein, Susan, and Giovanni Peri. 2018. "Immigrant Niches and Immigrant Networks in the US Labor Market." *Russell Sage Foundation Journal of the Social Sciences* 4 (1): 1–17.

Ehrenreich, Barbara, and Arlie R. Hochschild, eds. 2004. *Global Woman: Nannies, Maids, and Sex Workers in the New Economy.* New York: Henry Holt.

Emerson, Robert, and Melvin Pollner. 1976. "Dirty Work Designations: Their Features and Consequences in a Psychiatric Setting." *Social Problems* 23 (3): 243–254.

Emerson, Robert M., Rachel I. Fretz, and Linda L. Shaw. 2011. *Writing Ethnographic Field Notes.* Chicago: The University of Chicago Press.

England, Paula. 2005. "Emerging Theories of Care Work." *Annual Review of Sociology* 31 (1): 381–399.

England, Paula, Michelle Budig, and Nancy Folbre. 2002. "Wages of Virtue: The Relative Pay of Care Work." *Social Problems* 49 (4): 455–473.

Enriquez, Laura E. 2017a. "'A Master Status' or 'The Final Straw'? Assessing the Role of Immigration Status in Latino Undocumented Youths' Pathways Out of School." *Journal of Ethnic and Migration Studies* 43 (9): 1526–1543.

————. 2017b. "Gendering Illegality: Undocumented Young Adults' Negotiation of the Family Formation Process." *American Behavioral Scientist* 61 (10): 1153–1171.

————. 2020. *Of Love and Papers: How Immigration Policy Affects Romance and Family*. Berkeley: University of California Press.

Erickson, Rebecca, and Clare Stacey. 2013. "Attending to Mind and Body: Engaging the Complexity of Emotion Practice among Caring Professionals." In *Emotional Labor in the 21st Century: Diverse Perspectives on Emotion Regulation at Work*, edited by A. A. Grandey, J. M. Diefendorff, and D. E. Rupp. New York: Routledge.

Estrada, Emir. 2019. *Kids at Work: Latinx Families Selling Food on the Streets of Los Angeles*. New York: New York University Press.

Estrada, Emir, and Pierrette Hondagneu-Sotelo. 2013. "Living the Third Shift: Latina Adolescent Street Vendors in Los Angeles." In *Immigrant Workers in the Neoliberal Age*, edited by A. Guevarra, 144–163. Champaign, IL: University of Illinois Press.

Folbre, Nancy, ed. 2012. *For Love and Money: Care Provision in the United States*. New York: Russell Sage Foundation.

Folbre Nancy, Paula England, and Carrie Leana. 2012. "Motivating Care." In *For Love and Money: Care Provision in the United States*, edited by N. Folbre, 21–39. New York: Russell Sage Foundation.

Foner, Nancy. 1987. *New Immigrants in New York*. New York: Columbia University Press.

————. 1994. *The Caregiving Dilemma: Work in an American Nursing Home*. Berkeley: University of California Press.

Francisco-Menchavez, Valerie. 2018. *The Labor of Care: Filipina Migrants and Transnational Families in the Digital Age*. Urbana: University of Illinois Press.

Freed, Meredith, Juliette Cubanski, Tricia Neuman, Jennifer Klates, and Josh Michaud. 2020. "What Share of People Who Have Died of COVID-19 Are 65 and Older?—And How Does It Vary by State?" Kaiser Family Foundation. https://www.kff.org/coronavirus-covid-19/issue-brief/what-share-of-people-who-have-died-of-covid-19-are-65-and-older-and-how-does-it-vary-by-state/.

George, Sheba. 2005. *When Women Come First: Gender and Class in Transnational Migration*. Berkeley: University of California Press.

Gibson, Barbara, Nancy L. Young, Ross E. G. Upshur, and Patricia McKeever. 2007. "Men on the Margin: A Bourdieusian Examination of Living into Adulthood with Muscular Dystrophy." *Social Science and Medicine* 65:505–517.

Gillis, Catherine. 2010. "Making the Case for Nursing Workforce Diversity." *Nursing Outlook* 58 (5): 223–224.

Gleeson, Shannon, and Kati L. Griffith. 2020. "Employers as Subjects of the Immigration State: How State Security Foments Employment Security for Temporary Immigrant Workers." *Law and Social Inquiry* 46 (1): 92–115.

Glenn, Evelyn Nakano. 2010. *Forced to Care: Coercion and Caregiving in America*. Cambridge, MA: Harvard University Press.

Gonzales, Roberto G. 2016. *Lives in Limbo: Undocumented and Coming of Age in America*. Berkeley: University of California Press.

Gordon, April. 1998. "The New Diaspora—African Immigration to the United States" *Journal of Third World Studies* 15 (1).

Gottfried, Heide, and Jennifer Jiye Chun. 2018. "Care Work in Transition: Transnational Circuits of Gender, Migration, and Care." *Critical Sociology* 44 (7–8): 997–1012.

Government Accountability Office. 2020. "COVID-19: Urgent Actions Needed to Better Ensure an Effective Federal Response: Report to Congressional Committees (GAO-21-191)." https://www.gao.gov/products/GAO-21-191.

Gowayed, Heba. 2022. *Refuge: How the State Shapes Human Capital*. Princeton, NJ: Princeton University Press.

Guevarra, Anna. 2010. *Marketing Dreams, Manufacturing Heroes: The Transnational Labor Brokering of Filipino Workers*. New Brunswick, NJ: Rutgers University Press.

Gwaradzimba, Ellen, and Almon Shumba. 2010. "The Nature, Extent and Impact of the Brain Drain in Zimbabwe and South Africa." *Acta Academica* 42 (1): 209–241.

Habecker, Shelly. 2012. "Not Black but Habasha: Ethiopian and Eritrean Immigrants in American Society." *Ethnic and Racial Studies* 35 (7): 1200–1219.

Hagan, Jacqueline M., Rubén Hernández-León, and Jean-Luc Demonsant. 2015. *Skills of the "Unskilled:" Work and Mobility among Mexican Migrants*. Oakland: University of California Press.

Hall, Matthew, Emily Greenman, and Youngmin Yi. 2019. "Job Mobility and Unauthorized Immigrant Workers." *Social Forces* 97 (3): 999–1028.

Halter, Marilyn, and Violet Showers Johnson. 2014. *African and American: West African Immigrants in Post-Civil Rights America*. New York: New York University Press.

Hamilton, Tod. 2019. *Immigration and the Remaking of Black America*. New York: Russell Sage Foundation.

Hamilton, Tod, Janeria Easley, and Angela Dixon. 2018. "Black Immigration, Occupational Niches, and Earnings Disparities between U.S.-born and Foreign-Born Blacks in the United States." *Russel Sage Foundation Journal of the Social Sciences* 4:60–77.

Harrington-Meyer, Madonna, ed. 2000. *Care Work: Gender, Labor and the Welfare State*. New York: Routledge.

Harris-Kojetin, Lauren, Manisha Sengupta, Jessica P. Lendon, Vincent Rome, Roberto Valderde, and Christine Caffrey. 2019. "Long-Term Care Providers and Services Users in the United States, 2015–2016. National Center for Health Statistics." *Vital Health Stat* 3 (43).

Hefele, Jennifer Gaduet, Andrea Acevedo, Laurie Nsiah-Jefferson, Christine Bishop, Yasmin Abbas, Ecaterina Damien, and Candi Ramos. 2016. "Choosing a Nursing Home: What Do Consumers Want to Know and Do Preferences Vary across Race and Ethnicity?" *Health Services Research* 51 (2): 1167–1187.

Hine, Darlene Clark. 1989. *Black Women in White: Racial Conflict and Cooperation in the Nursing Profession, 1890–1950*. Bloomington: Indiana University Press.

Hochschild, Arlie. 1983. *The Managed Heart: Commercialization of Human Feeling*. Berkeley: University of California Press.

Holmes, Seth. 2013. *Fresh Fruit, Broken Bodies: Migrant Farmworkers in the United States*. Berkeley: University of California Press.

Hondagneu-Sotelo, Pierrette. 2001. *Doméstica: Immigrant Workers Cleaning and Caring in the Shadows of Affluence*. Berkeley: University of California Press.

Hooper, Kate, and Brian Salant. 2018. "It's Relative: A Cross-Country Comparison of Family-Migration Policies and Flows." https://www.migrationpolicy.org/research/crosscountry -comparison-family-migration.

Hughes, Everett. C. 1994. *On Work, Race, and the Sociological Imagination*. Chicago: University of Chicago Press.

Imoagene, Onoso. 2017. *Beyond Expectations: Second Generation Nigerians in the United States and Britain*. Berkeley: University of California Press.

Jackson, Regine. 2010. "Black Immigrants and the Rhetoric of Distancing." *Sociology Compass* 4 (3): 193–206.

Jacobs, Andrew. 2021. "Frontline Health Care Workers Aren't Feeling the 'Summer of Joy.'" *New York Times*. July 1. Updated August 26, 2021.

Jimenez, Tomas. 2017. *The Other Side of Assimilation: How Immigrants are Changing American Life*. Berkeley: University of California Press.

Kang, Miliann. 2010. *The Managed Hand: Race, Gender, and the Body in Beauty Service Work* Berkeley: University of California Press.

Kasinitz, Phillip, and Milton Vickerman. 2001. "Ethnic Niches and Racial Traps: Jamaicans in the New York Regional Economy." In *Migration, Transnationalization, & Race in a Changing New York*, edited by H. Cordero-Guzman, R. C. Smith, and R. Grosfoguel. Philadelphia: Temple University Press.

Kempadoo, Kamala.1999. *Sun, Sex, and Gold: Tourism and Sex Work in the Caribbean*. New York: Rowman and Littlefield.

Kibria, Nazli, Cara Bowman, and Megan O'Leary. 2014. *Race and Immigration*. Cambridge: Polity Press.

Kim, Dae Young. 2006. "Stepping-Stone to Intergenerational Mobility? The Springboard, Safety Net, or Mobility Trap Functions of Korean Immigrant Entrepreneurship for the Second Generation." *International Migration Review* 40 (4): 927–962.

Kingma, Mirielle. 2005. *Nurses on the Move: Migration and the Global Health Economy*. Ithaca, NY: Cornell University Press.

Konadu-Agyemang, Kwadwo, and Baffour K. Takyi. 2006. "Theoretical Perspectives on African Migration." In *The New African Diaspora in North America*, edited by K.-Konadu- Agyemang, B. K. Takyi, and J. Arthur. New York: Lexington Books.

Kowarski, Ilana. 2020 "How Coronavirus Affects Nursing School Admissions." US News. https://www.usnews.com/education/best-graduate-schools/top-nursing-schools /articles/how-coronavirus-is-affecting-nursing-school-admissions.

Lagasse, Jeff. 2020. "HealthCare Workers Experiencing Burnout, Stress Due to COVID-19 Pandemic." Healthcare Finance News (December 8). https://www.healthcarefinancenews .com/news/healthcare-workers-experiencing-burnout-stress-due-covid-19-pandemic.

Lamont. Michéle. 2000. *The Dignity of Working Men: Morality and the Boundaries of Race, Class, and Immigration*. New York: Russell Sage Foundation.

Lareau, Annette. 2003. *Unequal Childhoods: Race, Class and Family Life*. Berkeley: University of California Press.

LaVeist, Thomas A., Amani Nuru-Jeter, and Keisha. E. Jones. 2003. "The Association of Doctor-Patient Race Concordance with Health Care Services Utilization." *Journal of Public Health Policy* 24 (3–4): 312–323.

Lee, Jennifer, and Min Zhou. 2015. *The Asian American Achievement Paradox*. New York: Russell Sage Foundation.

Leidner, Robin. 1993. *Fast Food Fast Talk: Service Work and the Routinization of Everyday Life*. Berkeley: University of California Press.

Liang, Li-fang. 2011. "The Making of an 'Ideal' Live-In Migrant Care Worker: Recruiting, Training, Matching and Disciplining." *Ethnic and Racial Studies* 34 (11): 1815–1834.

Light, Ivan, and Steven J. Gold. 2000. *Ethnic Economies*. San Diego, CA: Academic Press.

Lofland, John, David Snow, Leon Anderson, and Lyn H. Lofland. 2006. *Analyzing Social Settings: A Guide to Qualitative Observation and Analysis*. Belmont, CA: Wadsworth.

Lopez, Steven. 2006. "Emotional Labor and Organized Emotional Care: Conceptualizing Nursing Home Care Work. *Work and Occupations* 33 (2): 133–360.

Lorenzi, Jane, and Jeanne Batalova. 2022. "Sub-Saharan African Immigrants in the United States." Migration Information Source, Migration Policy Institute. Retrieved June 21, 2022. https://www.migrationpolicy.org/article/sub-saharan-african-immigrants-united-states -2019.

Louie, Vivian. 2012. *Keeping the Immigrant Bargain: The Costs and Rewards of Success in America.* New York: Russell Sage Foundation.

Macdonald, Cameron. 2010. *Shadow Mothers: Nannies, Au Pairs, and the Micropolitics of Mothering.* Berkeley: University of California Press.

———. 2015. "Ethnic Logics: Race and Ethnicity in Nanny Employment." In *Caring on the Clock: The Complexities and Contradictions of Paid Care Work,* edited by M. Duffy, A. Armenia, and C. Stacey, 153–164. New Brunswick, NJ: Rutgers University Press.

Masselink, Leah E., and S. Y. Daniel Lee. 2010. "Nurses, Inc.: Expansion and Commercialization of Nursing Education in the Philippines. *Social Science & Medicine* 71:166–172.

Massey, Douglas. 1999. "Why Does Immigration Occur? A Theoretical Synthesis." In *Handbook of International Migration: The American Experience.* New York: Russell Sage Foundation.

Massey, Douglas, Margarita Mooney, Kimberly Torres, and Camille Charles. 2007. "Black Immigrants and Black Natives Attending Selective Colleges and Universities." *American Journal of Education* 113 (February): 243–271.

McCabe, Kristen. 2012. "African Immigrants in the United States." Migration Information Source, Migration Policy Institute. Retrieved May 15, 2013. http://www.migrationinformation.org/USFocus/display.cfm?ID=847.

McFadden, Patricia. 1997. "The Challenges and Prospects for the African Women's Movement in the 21st Century." *Women in Action,* no. 1.

McGarry, Brian E., David C. Grabowski, and Michael L. Barnett. 2020. "Severe Staffing and Personal Protective Equipment Shortages Faced by Nursing Homes during the COVID-19 Pandemic." *Health Affairs* 39 (10): 1–6.

McGregor, JoAnn. 2007. "Joining the BBC (British Bottom Cleaners): Zimbabwean Migrants and the UK Care Industry." *Journal of Ethnic and Migration Studies* 33 (5): 801–882.

Medford, Marcelle. 2019. "Racialization and Black Multiplicity: Generative Paradigms for Understanding Black Immigrants." *Sociology Compass* 13 (7): 1–16.

Meyer, Michelle, Michelle Donnelly, and Patricia Weerakoon. 2007. "'They're Taking the Place of My Hands': Perspectives of People Using Personal Care." *Disability & Society* 22 (6): 595–608.

Min, Pyong Gap. 2008. *Ethnic Solidarity for Economic Survival: Korean Greengrocers in New York City.* New York City: Russell Sage Foundation.

Miraftab, Faranak. 2016. *Global Heartland: Displaced Labor, Transnational Lives and Local Place Making.* Bloomington: Indiana University Press.

MITRE Corporation. 2020. Commission Final Report. Coronavirus Commission on Safety and Quality in Nursing Homes. McLean, VA. https://edit.cms.gov/files/document/covid-final-nh-commission-report.pdf.

Model, Suzanne. 2008. *West Indian Immigrants: A Black Success Story?* New York: Russell Sage Foundation.

Morgan, Jennifer Craft, Janette Dill, and Arne L. Kalleberg. 2013. "The Quality of Healthcare Jobs: Can Intrinsic Rewards Compensate for Low Extrinsic Rewards?" *Work, Employment and Society* 27 (5): 802–822.

Morrow, Lance. 1992. "Africa: The Scramble for Survival." *Time Magazine,* September 7.

Nazareno, Jennifer. 2018. "Welfare State Replacements: Deinstitutionalization, Privatization and the Outsourcing to Immigrant Women Enterprise." *International Journal of Health Services* 48 (2): 247–266.

Ong, Paul, and Tanya Azores. 1994. "The Migration and Incorporation of Philippines Nurses." In *The New Asian Immigration in Los Angeles and Global Restructuring,* edited by P. Ong, E. Bonacich, and L. Cheng, 164–195. Philadelphia: Temple University Press.

Ortiga, Yasmin Y. 2014. "Professional Problems: The Burden of Producing the 'Global' Filipino Nurse." *Social Science & Medicine* 115:64–71.

———. 2017. "The Flexible University: Higher Education and the Global Production of Migrant Labor." *British Journal of Sociology of Education* 38 (4): 485–499.

———. 2018. "Learning to Fill the Labor Niche: Filipino Nursing Graduates and the Risk of the Migration Trap." *Russell Sage Foundation Journal of the Social Sciences* 4 (1): 172–187.

Osirim, Mary Johnson. 2011. "Transnational Migration and Transformation among African Women in the United States: Change-Agents Locally and Globally." In *Analyzing Gender, Intersectionality, and Multiple Inequalities: Global, Transnational and Local Contexts*, edited by E. Chow, M. Segal, and L. Tan. Bingley, UK: Emerald Group.

———. 2012. "African Women in the New Diaspora: Transnationalism and the (Re)creation of Home." In *Africans in Global Migration*, edited by J. Arthur, J. Takougang, and T. Owusu. Lanham, MD: Lexington Books.

Osterman, Paul. 2017. *Who Will Care for Us? Long-Term Care and the Long-Term Workforce*. New York: Russell Sage Foundation.

Parreñas, Rhacel. 2001. *Servants of Globalization: Women, Migration and Domestic Work*. Stanford: Stanford University Press.

———. 2005. *Children of Global Migration: Transnational Families and Gendered Woes*. Stanford: Stanford University Press.

———. 2015. *Servants of Globalization: Women, Migration and Domestic Work* (2nd edition). Stanford: Stanford University Press.

Patler, Caitlin. 2018. "To Reveal or Conceal: How Diverse Undocumented Youth Navigate Legal Status Disclosure." *Sociological Perspectives* 61 (6): 857–873.

Patterson, Orlando. 2006. "A Poverty of Mind." *New York Times*. March 26.

Pearce, Susan, Elizabeth Clifford, and Reena Tandon. 2011. *Immigration and Women, Understanding the American Experience: Finding Agency, Negotiating Resistance and Bridging Cultures*. New York: New York University Press.

Pedraza, Silvia. 1991. "Women and Migration: The Social Consequences of Gender." *Annual Review of Sociology* 17: 303–325.

Phillips, Janice M., and Beverly Malone. 2014. "Increasing Racial/Ethnic Diversity in Nursing to Reduce Health Disparities and Achieve Health Equity." *Public Health Rep* Jan–Feb 29, (suppl 2): 45–50.

Pierre, Jemima. 2004. "Black Immigrants in the United States and the 'Cultural Narratives' of Ethnicity." *Identities: Global Studies in Culture and Power* 11 (2): 141–170.

Piore, Michael. 1979. *Birds of Passage*. Cambridge: Cambridge University Press.

Poros, Maritsa. 2011. *Modern Migrations: Gujarati Indian Networks in New York and London*. Stanford: Stanford University Press.

Portes, Alejandro, and Robert L. Bach. 1985. *Latin Journey: Cuban and Mexican Immigrants in the United States*. Berkeley and Los Angeles: University of California Press.

Portes, Alejandro, and Rubén Rumbaut. 2014. *Immigrant America: A Portrait*. Oakland: University of California Press.

Portes, Alejandro, and Min Zhou. 1993. "The New Second Generation: Segmented Assimilation and its Variants." *Annals of the American Academy of Political and Social Sciences* 530: 74–96.

Pradhan, Rachana, Lauren Weber, and Hannah Recht. 2020. "Lack of Antigen Test Reporting Leaves Country 'Blind to the Pandemic.'" Kaiser Health News. https://khn.org/news/lack-of-antigen-test-reporting-leaves-country-blind-to-the-pandemic/.

Prasad, Kristi, Collen McLoughlin, Martin Stillman, Sara Poplaw, Elizabeth Goelz, Sam Taylor, Nancy Nankivil, Roger Brown, Mark Linzer, Kyra Cappelucci, Michael Barbouche, and Christine A Sinsky. 2021. "Prevalence and Correlates of Stress and Burnout among U.S Healthcare Workers during the COVID-19 Pandemic: A National Cross-Sectional Study." *The Lancet* 35:100879. https://www.thelancet.com/journals/eclinm/article/PIIS2589 -5370(21)00159-0/fulltext.

Pratt, Geraldine. 1999. "From Registered Nurse to Registered Nanny: Discursive Geographies of Filipina Domestic Workers in Vancouver British Columbia." *Economic Geography* 75 (3): 215–236.

Purser, Gretchen. 2009. "The Dignity of Job-Seeking Men: Boundary Work among Immigrant Day Laborers." *Journal of Contemporary Ethnography* 38 (1): 117–139.

Raghuram, Parvati, and Eleonore Kofman. 2004. "Out of Asia: Skilling, Re-Skilling, and Deskilling of Female Immigrants." *Women's Studies International Forum* 27 (2): 95–100.

Rakovski, Carter, and Kim Price-Glynn. 2010. "Nursing Assistants, Caring Labor, and Intersectionality." *Sociology of Health & Illness* 32 (3): 400–414.

———. 2012. "Intersectional Identities and Worker Experiences in Home Health Care: The National Home Health Aide Survey." *Research in the Sociology of Health Care* 30: 261–280.

Ramirez, Hernan, and Pierrette Hondagneu-Sotelo. 2009. "Mexican Immigrant Gardeners: Entrepreneurs or Exploited Workers?" *Social Problems* 56 (1): 70–88.

Rodriguez, Robyn. 2010. *Migrants for Export: How the Philippine State Brokers Labor to the World*. Minneapolis: University of Minnesota Press.

Rodriguez, Robyn M., and Helen Schewenken. 2013. "Becoming a Migrant at Home: Subjectivation Processes in Migrant-Sending Countries Prior to Departure." *Population, Space and Place* 19 (4): 375–388.

Rodriquez, Jason. 2014. *Labors of Love: Nursing Homes and the Structures of Care Work*. New York: New York University Press.

Rollins, Judith. 1987. *Between Women: Domestics and their Employers*. Philadelphia: Temple University Press.

Rosales, Rocío. 2020. *Fruteros: Street Vending, Illegality, and Ethnic Community in Los Angeles*. Oakland: University of California Press.

Rothenberg, Daniel. 2000. *With These Hands: The Hidden World of Migrant Farm Workers Today*. Berkeley: University of California Press.

Ruchti, Lisa C. 2012. *Catheters, Slurs and Pickup Lines: Professional Intimacy in Hospital Nursing*. Philadelphia: Temple University Press.

Sacks, Tina K. 2019. *Invisible Visits: Black Middle-Class Women in the American Health Care System*. Oxford: Oxford University Press.

Safa, Helen. 1995. *The Myth of the Male Bread Winner: Women and Industrialization in the Caribbean*. Boulder, CO: Westview Press.

Sanders, Jimy M., and Victor Nee. 1996. "Immigrant Self-Employment: The Family as Social Capital and the Value of Human Capital." *American Sociological Review* 61 (2): 231–249.

Sassen, Saskia. 1991. *The Global City: New York, London, Tokyo*. Princeton, NJ: Princeton University Press.

Schweid, Richard. 2021. *The Caring Class: Home Health Aides in Crisis*. Ithaca, NY: Cornell University Press.

Scrinzi, Francesca. 2010. "Masculinities and the International Division of Care: Migrant Male Domestic Workers in Italy and France." *Men and Masculinities* 13 (1): 44–64.

Showers, Fumilayo. 2015a. "Being Black, Foreign and Woman: African Immigrant Identities in the United States." *Ethnic and Racial Studies* 38 (10): 1815–30.

———. 2015b. "Building a Professional Identity: Boundary Work and Meaning-Making among West African Immigrant Nurses." In *Caring on the Clock: The Complexities and Con-*

traditions of Paid Care Work, edited by M. Duffy, A. Armenia, and C. Stacey, 143–152. New Brunswick, NJ: Rutgers University Press.

———. 2018. "Learning to Care: Work Experiences and Identity Formation among African Immigrant Care Workers." *International Journal of Care and Caring* 2 (1): 7–25.

Showers Johnson, Violet. 2008. "'What, Then, Is the African American?' African and Afro-Caribbean Identities in Black America." *Journal of American Ethnic History* 28 (1): 77–103.

Smith, Robert. C. 2006. *Mexican New York: Transnational Lives of the New Immigrants*. Berkeley: University of California Press.

Solari, Cinzia. 2006. "Professionals and Saints: How Immigrant Care Workers Negotiate Gender Identities at Work." *Gender & Society* 20:301.

Squires, Allison, and H. Beltran Sanchez. 2013. "Strengthening Health Systems in North and Central America: What Role for Migration?" Retrieved November 2, 2020. https://www.migrationpolicy.org/research/strengthening-health-systems-north-and-central-america-what-role-migration.

Stacey, Clare. 2005. "Finding Dignity in Dirty Work: The Constraints and Rewards of Low-Wage Home Care Labour." *Sociology of Health and Illness* 27 (6): 831–854.

———. 2011. *The Caring Self: The Work Experiences: of Home Care Aides*. Ithaca, NY: Cornell University Press.

Stoller, Paul. 2001. *Money Has No Smell: The Africanization of New York City*. Chicago: University of Chicago Press.

Strauss, Anselm, and Juliet J. Corbin. 1994. "Grounded Theory Methodology." In *Handbook of Qualitative Research*, edited by N. K. Denzin and Y. S. Lincoln, 273–285. Thousand Oaks, CA: Sage.

Suárez Orozco, Marcelo M., and Carola Suárez Orozco. 1995. "The Cultural Patterning of Achievement Motivation: A Comparative Study of Mexican, Mexican Immigrant, and Non-Latino White American Youths in Schools." In *California's Immigrant Children: Theory, Research, and Implications for Educational Policy*, edited by R. Rumbaut and W. Cornelius, 161–190. La Jolla: Center for U.S.-Mexican Studies, University of California San Diego.

Talaee Negin, Mohammad Varahram, Hamidreza Jamaati, Alireza Salimi, Mirsaeed Attarchi, Mehdi Kazempour Dizaji, Makan Sadr, Somayeh Hassani, Behrooz Farzanegan, Fateme Monjazebi, and Seyed Mohammad Seyedmehdi. 2020. "Stress and Burnout in Health Care Workers during COVID-19 Pandemic: Validation of a Questionnaire." *Zeitschrift fur Gesundheitswissenschaften (Journal of Public Health)* 6:1–6.

Tesfai, Rebecca. 2019. "Double Minority Status and Neighborhoods: Examining the Primacy of Race in Black Immigrants Racial and Socioeconomic Segregation." *City and Community* 18 (2): 509–528.

———. 2020. "Immigrants' Occupational Segregation in France: 'Brown-Collar' Jobs or a Sub-Saharan African Disadvantage?" *Ethnic and Racial Studies* 43 (15): 2724–2745.

———. 2021. "Is There any Merit to the Merit-Based Immigration System? What Sub-Saharan African Immigrant Labor and Housing Market Outcomes Tell Us about U.S. Economic and Immigration Systems." *Sociology Compass* 15 (5). https://doi.org/10.1111/soc4.12873.

Tesfai, Rebecca, and Kevin J. A. Thomas. 2020. "Dimensions of Inequality: Black Immigrants' Occupational Segregation in the United States." *Sociology of Race and Ethnicity* 6 (1): 1–21.

Thomas, Kevin J. A. 2014. *Diverse Pathways: Race and the Incorporation of Black, White, and Arab-Origin Africans in the United States*. East Lansing: Michigan State University Press.

Twigg, Julia. 1999. "The Spatial Ordering of Care: Public and Private in Bathing Support at Home." *Sociology of Health and Illness* 4 (2): 381–400.

———. 2000. *Bathing: The Body and Community Care*. London: Routledge.

Ungerson, Clare. 1999. "Personal Assistants and Disabled People: An Examination of a Hybrid Form of Work and Care." *Work, Employment, & Society* 13 (4): 583–600.

Valdez, Zulema. 2008. "The Effect of Social Capital on Korean, White, Mexican, and Black Business Owners' Earnings." *Journal of Ethnic and Migration Studies* 34 (6): 955–974.

———. 2011. *The New Entrepreneurs: How Race, Class, and Gender Shape Entrepreneurship*. Stanford: Stanford University Press.

Vallejo, Jody Aguis, and Stephanie L. Canizales. 2016. "Latino Professionals as Entrepreneurs: How Race, Class, and Gender Shape Entrepreneurial Incorporation." *Ethnic and Racial Studies* 39 (9): 1637–1656.

Van Houtven, Carol Harold, Nicole DePasquale, and Norma B. Coe. 2020. "Essential Long-Term Care Workers Commonly Hold Second Jobs and Double- or Triple-Duty Caregiving Roles." *Journal of the American Geriatrics Society* 68 (8): 1657–1660.

Veit, Susanne, and Lex Thijsen. 2021. "Almost Identical but Still Treated Differently: Hiring Discrimination against Foreign-Born and Domestic-Born Minorities." *Journal of Ethnic and Migration Studies* 47 (6): 1285–1304.

Verdaguer, Maria. 2009. *Class, Ethnicity, Gender and Latino Entrepreneurship*. New York: Routledge Publishing.

Vickerman, Milton. 1999. *Crosscurrents: West Indian Immigrants and Race*. Oxford: Oxford University Press.

———. 2001. "Tweaking a Monolith: The West Indian Immigrant Encounter with Blackness." In *Islands in the City*, edited by N. Foner, 237–256. Los Angeles: University of California Press.

———. 2007. "Recent Immigration and Race." *Dubois Review: Social Science Research on Race* 4 (1): 141–165.

Waldinger, Roger. 1994. "The Making of an Immigrant Niche." *International Migration Review* 28 (1): 3–30.

———. 1996. *Still the Promised City? New Immigrants and African Americans in Post-Industrial New York*. Cambridge, MA: Harvard University Press.

Waldinger, Roger, and Michael Lichter. 2003. *How the Other Half Works*. Berkeley: University of California Press.

Walton-Roberts, Margaret. 2012. "Contextualizing the Global Nursing Care Chain: International Migration and the Status of Nursing in Kerala, India." *Global Networks* 12 (2): 175–194.

———. 2015. "International Migration of Health Professionals and the Marketization and Privatization of Health Education in India: From Push-Pull to Global Political Economy." *Social Science & Medicine* 124:374–382.

Waters, Mary C. 2001. *Black Identities: West Indian Immigrant Dreams and American Realities*. Cambridge, MA: Harvard University Press.

———. 1990. *Ethnic Options: Choosing Identities in America*. Berkeley: University of California Press.

Weber, Lauren. 2021. "Nursing Homes Keep Losing Workers." *Wall Street Journal*, August 25.

Williams, Christine. 1991. *Gender Differences at Work: Women and Men in Nontraditional Occupations*. Berkeley: University of California Press.

Williams, Joseph P. 2021. "Strapped by Shortages and Hit with Departures, Nurse Corps Swamped by Another COVID Wave." US News, August 19. https://www.usnews.com/news/health-news/articles/2021-08-19/fourth-covid-wave-swamps-stressed-nurse-corps.

Wingfield, Adia Harvey. 2019. *Flatlining: Race, Work and Health Care in the New Economy*. Oakland: University of California Press.

————. 2009. "Racializing the Glass Escalator: Reconsidering Men's Experiences with Women's Work." *Gender and Society* 23 (1): 5–26.

Wingfield, Adia, and Koji Chavez. 2020. "Getting In, Getting Hired, Getting Sideways Looks: Organizational Hierarchy and Perceptions of Workplace Racial Discrimination." *American Sociological Review* 85 (1): 31–57.

Yeates, Nicola. 2009. *Globalizing Care Economies and Migrant Workers: Explorations in Global Care Chains*. London: Palgrave Macmillan.

Zeleza, Paul. 2009. "Diaspora Dialogues: Engagements between Africa and its Diaspora." In *The New African Diaspora*, edited by I. Opkewho and N. Zwegu, 31–58. Bloomington: Indiana University Press.

Zelizer, Viviana. 2005. *The Purchase of Intimacy*. Princeton, NJ: Princeton University Press.

Zhou, Min, and Carl L. Bankston III. 1998. *Growing Up American: How Vietnamese Children Adapt to Life in the United States*. New York: Russell Sage Foundation.

Zimmerman, Mary K., Jacqueline S. Litt, and Christine E. Bose, eds. 2006. *Global Dimensions of Gender and Care Work*. Stanford: Stanford University Press.

Zong, Jie, and Jeanne Batalova. 2017. "Sub-Saharan African Immigrants in the United States." Washington, DC: Migration Policy Institute. https://www.migrationpolicy.org/article/sub-saharan-african-immigrants-united-states-2015.

INDEX

ABOUT THE AUTHOR

FUMILAYO SHOWERS is assistant professor of sociology and Africana studies at the University of Connecticut.